CONTENTS

INTRODUCTION

PasTest's MRCP Part 1 Pocket Books are designed to help the busy examination candidate to make the most of every opportunity to revise. With this little book in your pocket, it is the work of a moment to open it, choose a question, decide upon your answers and then check the answer. Revising 'on the run' in this manner is both reassuring (if your answer is correct) and stimulating (if you find any gaps in your knowledge).

The MRCP Part 1 examination consists of two papers, each lasting three hours. Both papers contain 100 'Best of Five' questions (one answer is chosen from five options). Questions in each specialty are randomised across both papers. *No marks are deducted for a wrong answer.*

One-best answer/'Best of Five' MCQs
An important characteristic of one-best answer MCQs is that they can be designed to test application of knowledge and clinical problem-solving rather than just the recall of facts. This should change (for the better) the ways in which candidates prepare for MRCP Part 1.

Each one-best MCQ has a question stem, which usually contains clinical information, followed by five branches. All five branches are typically homologous (eg all diagnoses, all laboratory investigations, all antibiotics) and should be set out in a logical order (eg alphabetical). Candidates are asked to select the ONE branch that is the best answer to the question. A response is not required to the other four branches. The answer sheet is, therefore, slightly different to that used for true/false MCQs.

A good strategy that can be used with many well-written one-best MCQs is to try to reach the correct answer without first scrutinising the five options. If you can then find the answer you have reached in the option list, then you are probably correct.

One-best answer MCQs are quicker to answer than multiple true/false MCQs because only one response is needed for each question. Even though the question stem for one-best answer MCQs is usually longer than for true/false questions, and therefore takes a little longer to read carefully, it is reasonable to set more one-best than true/false MCQs for the same exam duration – in this instance 60 true/false and 100 one-best are used in exams of two hours' duration.

Application of Knowledge and Clinical Problem-Solving
Unlike true/false MCQs, which test mainly the recall of knowledge, one-best answer questions test application and problem-solving. This makes them more effective test items and is one of the reasons why testing time can be reduced. In order to answer

these questions correctly, it is necessary to apply basic knowledge – not just be able to remember it. Furthermore, candidates who cannot reach the correct answer by applying their knowledge are much less likely to be able to choose the right answer by guessing than they were with true/false MCQs. This gives a big advantage to the best candidates, who have good knowledge and can apply it in clinical situations.

Books like the ones in this series, which consist of 'Best of Five' questions in subject categories, can help you to focus on specific topics and to isolate your weaknesses. You should plan a revision timetable to help you spread your time evenly over the range of subjects likely to appear in the examination. PasTest's *Essential Revision Notes for MRCP* by P Kalra will provide you with essential notes on all aspects of the syllabus.

CONTRIBUTORS

SECOND EDITION

Clinical Pharmacology

Professor M Pirmohamed PhD FRCP FRCP (Edin) Professor of Clinical Pharmacology and Hon Consultant Physician, Department of Pharmacology and Therapeutics, University of Liverpool, Liverpool.

Immunology

Neil Snowden FRCP FRCPath Consultant Rheumatologist, North Manchester General Hospital, Manchester.

Alan J Hakim MA MRCP, Consultant Rheumatologist and General Physician, Whipp's Cross University Hospital, London, Honorary Consultant Rheumatologist, University College London Hospitals.

Infectious Diseases

Ian Cropley MA MBBS MRCP Consultant in Infectious Diseases and HIV, Royal Free Hospital, London

Alan J Hakim MA MRCP, Consultant Rheumatologist and General Physician, Whipp's Cross University Hospital, London, Honorary Consultant Rheumatologist University College London Hospitals

Rheumatology

Anne Barton MRCP PhD MSc BSc(Hons) Consultant Rheumatologist and Clinical Lecturer, East Cheshire NHS Trust and University of Manchester

Alan J Hakim MA MRCP, Consultant Rheumatologist and General Physician, Whipp's Cross University Hospital, London, Honorary Consultant Rheumatologist University College London Hospitals

FIRST EDITION

Clinical Pharmacology

Professor M Pirmohamed PhD FRCP FRCP (Edin) Professor of Clinical Pharmacology and Hon Consultant Physician, Department of Pharmacology and Therapeutics, University of Liverpool, Liverpool.

Immunology

Alan J Hakim MA MRCP, Consultant Rheumatologist and General Physician, Whipp's Cross University Hospital, London, Honorary Consultant Rheumatologist University College London Hospitals

Infectious Diseases

Alan J Hakim MA MRCP, Consultant Rheumatologist and General Physician, Whipp's Cross University Hospital, London, Honorary Consultant Rheumatologist University College London Hospitals

Rheumatology

Alan J Hakim MA MRCP, Consultant Rheumatologist and General Physician, Whipp's Cross University Hospital, London, Honorary Consultant Rheumatologist University College London Hospitals.

CLINICAL PHARMACOLOGY

Best of Five

Questions

CLINICAL PHARMACOLOGY: 'BEST OF FIVE' QUESTIONS

For each of the questions select the ONE most appropriate answer from the options provided.

1.1 A 76-year-old man presents with bacterial conjunctivitis. The GP prescribes an antibiotic whose mode of action is through inhibition of protein synthesis. Which one of the following antibiotics did he prescribe?

- ☐ A Chloramphenicol
- ☐ B Penicillin
- ☐ C Ciprofloxacin
- ☐ D Rifampicin
- ☐ E Teicoplanin

1.2 A 23-year-old patient presents with a polyuria, polydipsia and weight loss and is diagnosed as having insulin-dependent diabetes mellitus (IDDM). Which one of the following facts should be taken into consideration in the management of this patient?

- ☐ A Effective control of blood sugar has been shown to decrease long-term complications
- ☐ B Insulin lispro has a slower onset of action than soluble insulin
- ☐ C Insulin lispro lowers glycosylated haemoglobin
- ☐ D Porcine insulin is less immunogenic than human insulin
- ☐ E Patients should reduce their insulin dosage if they develop an intercurrent infection

1.3 A 60-year-old woman is diagnosed with breast cancer. She has a lumpectomy and is started on tamoxifen 20 mg per day. Which one of the following is true with regard to the use of tamoxifen in breast cancer?

- ☐ A It is more effective in pre-menopausal women with breast cancer than in post-menopausal women
- ☐ B It is known to reduce the risk of endometrial cancer
- ☐ C It can cause retinopathy
- ☐ D It can result in hypocalcaemia
- ☐ E It is a pure antagonist at oestrogen receptors

1.4   A 28-year-old homosexual man with a diagnosis of HIV infection is started on protease inhibitor in combination with abacavir and lamivudine for treatment. The physician counsels him and warns him about the possible occurrence of lipodystrophy with protease inhibitors. Lipodystrophy caused by protease inhibitors is characterised by which one of the following?

- ☐ A   Hypoglycaemia
- ☐ B   Insulin resistance
- ☐ C   Uveitis
- ☐ D   Peripheral neuropathy
- ☐ E   Renal failure

1.5   You are in charge of an antenatal clinic and are frequently consulted by midwives in relation to the possible teratogenic effects of drugs being taken by pregnant women. Which one of the following drugs has been proved to have teratogenic effects in pregnant women?

- ☐ A   Diazepam
- ☐ B   Misoprostol
- ☐ C   Heparin
- ☐ D   Oral contraceptives
- ☐ E   Aspirin

1.6   A 50-year-old woman consults you about the possibility of starting hormone replacement therapy (HRT). You discuss the benefits and risks of HRT. Which one of the following statements regarding HRT is true?

- ☐ A   Unopposed oestrogens should not be used in patients who have had a hysterectomy
- ☐ B   It is associated with a twofold increased risk of breast cancer
- ☐ C   Conventional forms of hormone replacement therapy are less effective than newer compounds such as raloxifene
- ☐ D   Its use increases the risk of Alzheimer's disease
- ☐ E   The benefits on bone are the same irrespective of when the drugs are started after the menopause

1.7   A 27-year-old woman presents with an overdose of a number of drugs which she has taken from the bathroom cabinet at home. Which one of the following is the most important consideration in her management?

☐ A   Gastric lavage should be used up to six hours after the overdose

☐ B   Ipecacuanha syrup should be used routinely

☐ C   Activated charcoal reduces the enterohepatic circulation of drugs

☐ D   Haemodialysis is useful for eliminating drugs with a high volume of distribution

☐ E   Alkalinisation of urine should be used in all patients who have taken an aspirin overdose

1.8   You are asked to see a 30-year-old woman with hypertension who has peculiar dietary habits. In particular, she drinks two litres of grapefruit juice per day. You are concerned that this may lead to a serious interaction with which one of the following drugs that she is taking?

☐ A   Perindopril

☐ B   Ciclosporin

☐ C   Atenolol

☐ D   Bendroflumethiazide (bendrofluazide)

☐ E   Sodium valproate

1.9   A 70-year-old man presents with depression which you feel needs drug treatment. You choose to use fluoxetine but the product information reveals that it undergoes extensive drug metabolism. Which one of the following statements concerning the process of drug metabolism is correct?

☐ A   The primary role of drug metabolism is to convert hydrophilic compounds into lipophilic compounds

☐ B   Drugs are only metabolised in the liver

☐ C   Metabolism leads to the inactivation of fluoxetine

☐ D   Cytochrome P450 enzymes are largely responsible for the phase II metabolic pathways

☐ E   Genetically determined deficiencies of some of the drug metabolising enzymes have been described

1.10 A 20-year-old man presents with symptoms of schizophrenia. In deciding on which drug to use, you consider that atypical neuroleptics in comparison to typical neuroleptics are generally:

- ☐ A Less likely to cause parkinsonism
- ☐ B More likely to cause neuroleptic malignant syndrome
- ☐ C Less likely to affect the negative symptoms of schizophrenia
- ☐ D Less likely to affect the positive symptoms of schizophrenia
- ☐ E Less likely to cause weight gain

1.11 A two-year-old child develops infantile spasms and is started on vigabatrin by the paediatric neurologist. The mode of action of vigabatrin is thought to be through which one of the following?

- ☐ A Glutamate antagonism
- ☐ B Inhibition of GABA re-uptake
- ☐ C Inhibition of calcium conductance
- ☐ D Inhibition of sodium conductance
- ☐ E Inhibition of GABA transaminase

1.12 A 30-year-old man with bipolar depression is started on lithium carbonate. Which one of the following actions does this drug have?

- ☐ A It affects mood in normal subjects
- ☐ B It can cause central diabetes insipidus
- ☐ C It interacts with bendroflumethiazide (bendrofluazide)
- ☐ D It can be used in breastfeeding mothers
- ☐ E It can be used without dose alteration in patients with moderate to severe renal impairment

1.13 A 46-year-old man develops an acute attack of gout which is treated with high-dose diclofenac. Which one of the following drugs may be used safely in this patient without any risk of precipitating gout?

- ☐ A Allopurinol
- ☐ B Probenecid
- ☐ C Atenolol
- ☐ D Adenosine
- ☐ E Ciclosporin

1.14 **On a typical infectious diseases ward round you see many patients with different infections and on a variety of antibiotics. Regarding the use of antibiotics, which one of the following is a known characteristic?**

☐ A   Clindamycin is not used in the treatment of osteomyelitis because it does not penetrate bone well

☐ B   Clindamycin can be used for the treatment of pseudomembranous colitis

☐ C   Co-amoxiclav is effective against methicillin-resistant *Staphylococcus aureus*

☐ D   Amoxicillin is well known to cause cholestatic hepatitis

☐ E   Clarithromycin is active against atypical mycobacteria

1.15 **You have just taken over a primary care practice and are told of the very high drugs bill of the practice compared with other local comparator practices. While going through drug records, you notice that many patients are on branded products despite the availability of similar generic drugs. You present your findings at a meeting and suggest that patients should be changed to generic drugs. This leads to a debate and you are asked various questions about generic drugs. Which one of the following statements is true?**

☐ A   Demonstration of bioequivalence with the brand leader is not usually required before the drug is allowed to be marketed

☐ B   Bioequivalence with modified-release preparations is readily demonstrable

☐ C   Bioequivalence studies are usually single-dose studies

☐ D   Bioequivalence studies are performed in patients with the relevant diseases

☐ E   Different brands of prednisolone vary widely in bioavailability and must be prescribed by brand name

1.16 As part of a new post in a teaching hospital you are asked to give a lecture on pharmacokinetics. Which one of the following statements regarding pharmacokinetics is correct?

☐ A A first-pass effect means that a drug only works the first time it is taken

☐ B Zero-order kinetics means that the rate of elimination of the drug is dependent on the plasma concentration

☐ C Bioavailability refers to the percentage of drug being excreted by the kidneys

☐ D The terminal half-life of a drug is the time taken to excrete all of a given dose

☐ E Glucuronidation usually increases the lipid-solubility of a drug

1.17 A 75-year-old woman on digoxin presents to the Emergency Department with nausea, vomiting and palpitations, which you feel may be due to digoxin toxicity. Which one of the following statements regarding digoxin toxicity is true?

☐ A It is potentiated by hypocalcaemia

☐ B It is potentiated by hyponatraemia

☐ C It is diagnosed by ST elevation on an ECG

☐ D It is treated with phenytoin

☐ E It is treated with an infusion of calcium chloride

1.18 A 72-year-old man is diagnosed with motor neurone disease and is started on riluzole. Which one of the following is a known feature of riluzole?

☐ A It acts as a glutamate agonist

☐ B It can only be used in amyotrophic lateral sclerosis

☐ C It improves functional capacity in patients with amyotrophic lateral sclerosis

☐ D It causes an increase in liver enzymes in more than 1 in 1000 patients

☐ E It has been shown to improve quality of life

1.19 A 68-year-old lady from Kenya presents with anaemia which you consider to be caused by the number of drugs she is currently taking. Which one of the following drugs is not usually a cause of anaemia?

☐ A   Metformin

☐ B   Meloxicam

☐ C   Alendronate

☐ D   Atenolol

☐ E   Nitrofurantoin

1.20 On a routine ward round you come across a 30-year-old diabetic patient on several drugs which you think act via receptors. Which one of the following is correct regarding receptor action?

☐ A   Receptors are present only on the plasma membrane

☐ B   Receptors initiate the pharmacological actions of all drugs

☐ C   Receptor actions remain constant in the continued presence of an agonist

☐ D   Receptors interacting with G proteins usually stimulate guanylate cyclase activity

☐ E   Insulin receptors are linked to transmembrane protein tyrosine kinases

1.21 A 45-year-old man presents with epigastric pain and is diagnosed as having a duodenal ulcer on endoscopy. Biopsy of the duodenum shows the presence of *Helicobacter pylori*. Which one of the following statements is true regarding infection of the stomach by *Helicobacter pylori*?

☐ A   There is no need to eradicate *H. pylori* in patients with peptic ulcer

☐ B   Patients with non-specific dyspepsia have been shown to benefit from eradication therapy

☐ C   Long-term therapy with omeprazole without antibiotics can alter the distribution of infection within the stomach

☐ D   The different eradication therapies are generally associated with an eradication rate of 70%

☐ E   It is associated with an increase risk of cancer of the duodenum

1.22   **A 27-year-old with a long history of intravenous drug use presents with increased transaminases. He is diagnosed as being hepatitis C-positive and the hepatologist decides to use interferon-α and ribavarin for treatment. Which one of the following is true regarding the use of interferon-α in chronic hepatitis C virus infection?**

- ☐ A   A sustained response rate is seen in 50% of patients
- ☐ B   Fever is a rare adverse effect
- ☐ C   It can lead to bone marrow suppression
- ☐ D   Response is better in patients who are currently abusing alcohol
- ☐ E   The concomitant use of paracetamol is contraindicated

1.23   **A 32-year-old diabetic woman presents with proteinuria and you feel that she would benefit from either an angiotensin-II receptor antagonist or an angiotensin-converting enzyme (ACE) inhibitor. Which one of the following properties do these two groups of drugs share?**

- ☐ A   They cause cough as an adverse effect
- ☐ B   They have a similar incidence of angio-oedema
- ☐ C   They cause blockade of the degradation of bradykinin
- ☐ D   They are contraindicated in patients with bilateral renal artery stenosis
- ☐ E   They can be used safely in patients with pregnancy-induced hypertension

1.24   **A ten-year-old boy presents with fever and purpuric rash and is quickly diagnosed as having meningococcal meningitis. Which one of the following is true regarding the treatment of meningococcal meningitis?**

- ☐ A   Treatment should be withheld until cultures are taken in patients with suspected disease
- ☐ B   Dexamethasone should be routinely administered in patients with septicaemia
- ☐ C   Chemoprophylaxis is indicated for intimate but not household contacts
- ☐ D   Chemoprophylaxis is indicated for all health-care workers coming into contact with the patient
- ☐ E   Treatment with ceftriaxone is superior to treatment with cefuroxime

1.25   A 27-year-old woman presents to the Emergency Department after taking 48 Anadin® tablets. Which one of the following symptoms would you expect to find in this patient?

☐ A   Tinnitus

☐ B   Hyperglycaemia

☐ C   Metabolic alkalosis

☐ D   Peptic ulceration

☐ E   Hypercoagulability

1.26   A 20-year-old schizophrenic patient is started on chlorpromazine. He presents four weeks later feeling unwell and is diagnosed as having neuroleptic malignant syndrome. Which one of the following statements is true regarding neuroleptic malignant syndrome?

☐ A   It is a dose-related adverse effect of phenothiazines

☐ B   Affected patients are fully conscious

☐ C   Calcium-channel blockers have been shown to reduce mortality

☐ D   It is characterised by elevated troponin T levels

☐ E   It has an insidious onset

1.27   A 68-year-old man presents with acute atrial fibrillation. Which one of the following is true regarding the treatment of atrial fibrillation?

☐ A   Adenosine is beneficial in the treatment of atrial fibrillation

☐ B   Digoxin should be the first-line therapy in paroxysmal atrial fibrillation

☐ C   Sotalol has class II (β-blocking) effects only

☐ D   Propafenone has α-adrenoceptor-blocking activity

☐ E   Magnesium may be of use in patients with rapid atrial fibrillation

1.28   You are asked to perform an audit on drug-drug interactions. On reviewing your notes you come up with the following combinations that were prescribed in patients. Which one of the following combinations would you consider to be harmful?

☐ A   Rifabutin and clarithromycin

☐ B   Zidovudine and aciclovir

☐ C   Isosorbide mononitrate and atenolol

☐ D   Aspirin and streptokinase

☐ E   Naproxen and penicillamine

1.29   A 26-year-old epileptic patient on carbamazepine develops toxic epidermal necrolysis which necessitates intensive treatment on ITU and a six-week hospital stay. You decide to report this reaction on a yellow adverse drug reaction (ADR) reporting form. Which one of the following statements regarding ADR reporting in the UK is correct?

☐   A   ADR reporting is compulsory

☐   B   All serious ADRs should be reported

☐   C   A black triangle (▼) sign by a drug in the *British National Formulary* (BNF) indicates that only allergic reactions need be reported

☐   D   Only doctors, dentists and coroners are allowed to report on yellow cards

☐   E   Yellow card reports allow a causal relationship to be established between a drug and an ADR

1.30   A 30-year-old man who weighs 70 kg presents with a large aspirin overdose. Haemodialysis is a treatment modality, the success of which will depend on the apparent volume of distribution (Vd). Which one of the following statements about Vd is correct in this man?

☐   A   Vd does not exceed the volume of total body water

☐   B   Vd would be expected to be 25 litres if the drug remained in the blood

☐   C   Overdose of a drug with a high Vd can be treated by haemodialysis

☐   D   Vd is low if the drug is avidly bound in the tissues

☐   E   Vd can be calculated from a knowledge of the dose and concentration in plasma if the drug demonstrates linear kinetics

1.31   Pyridoxine (vitamin B_6) is a widely used vitamin in conditions such as premenstrual syndrome. It is also abused by body builders. Which one of the following is a known characteristic of pyridoxine?

☐   A   Vitamin B_6 status can be assessed by the tryptophan loading test

☐   B   Prolonged use of penicillin can lead to vitamin B_6 deficiency

☐   C   Its use is contraindicated in pregnant women

☐   D   It should not be given to patients with Parkinson's disease being treated with co-careldopa (L-dopa and carbidopa)

☐   E   It is excreted unchanged by the kidneys

1.32   A 20-year-old lady presents with weight loss, tremor, sweating and a goitre. A clinical diagnosis of thyrotoxicosis is made and is confirmed by a suppressed TSH level. Which one of the following is true regarding the use of antithyroid drugs?

  ☐ A   Carbimazole inhibits the peripheral conversion of T_4 to T_3

  ☐ B   β-Blockers reduce the basal metabolic rate

  ☐ C   Carbimazole produces an improvement in two days

  ☐ D   Iodide can cause a goitre in euthyroid patients

  ☐ E   Radioactive iodine (^{131}I) predominantly emits γ rays

1.33   A 26-year-old man presents with methanol poisoning. Which one of the following is a known feature of poisoning with methanol?

  ☐ A   The major route of elimination of methanol is via the kidneys

  ☐ B   Optic atrophy occurs within a few days

  ☐ C   Monitoring of blood levels is not required

  ☐ D   Metabolic acidosis with a normal anion gap is the usual finding

  ☐ E   Ethanol prevents methanol toxicity by inhibiting its oxidation within the liver

1.34   A 40-year-old alcoholic man presents to your clinic complaining of the recent onset of flushing when alcohol is consumed. Which one of the following drugs is most likely to be responsible for this adverse effect?

  ☐ A   Propranolol

  ☐ B   Chlorpromazine

  ☐ C   Thiamine

  ☐ D   Metronidazole

  ☐ E   Naltrexone

1.35 A recent report from the House of Lords warned against the overuse of antibiotics, particularly in primary medicine. Recent data suggest that resistance to penicillins is present in 20% or more of isolates of which one of the following bacterial species?

- [ ] A *Escherichia coli*
- [ ] B *Neisseria meningitidis*
- [ ] C Beta-haemolytic streptococci
- [ ] D *Streptococcus pneumoniae*
- [ ] E *Haemophilus influenzae*

1.36 Your hospital is drawing up new guidelines for the management of patients admitted with venous thromboembolism. One area for consideration is the use of low molecular weight heparins instead of unfractionated heparin. Low molecular weight heparins in comparison to unfractionated heparin are:

- [ ] A Weaker inhibitors of thrombin
- [ ] B Less likely to have reduced clearance in patients with renal failure
- [ ] C Less likely to cause bleeding
- [ ] D More likely to cause thrombocytopenia
- [ ] E More likely to cause osteoporosis during long-term administration

1.37 A 70-year-old woman presents with breast cancer. After surgery the patient is started on an aromatase inhibitor. Which one of the following is true regarding the use of aromatase inhibitors?

- [ ] A Anastrazole is a less potent inhibitor than aminoglutethimide
- [ ] B Corticosteroid replacement is necessary in patients on aminoglutethimide
- [ ] C Anastrazole affects adrenal function
- [ ] D They are efficacious in pre- and post-menopausal women
- [ ] E Inhibition of aromatase occurs predominantly within the ovaries rather than in extraglandular sites

1.38 A 45-year-old man with a body mass index of 33 kg/m^2 has failed to lose weight on various diet and exercise programmes and is considered for anti-obesity drug therapy. Which one of the following statements regarding obesity and its treatment is correct?

☐ A Sibutramine can be used in patients with hypertension

☐ B Heart valve regurgitation has been shown to be associated with treatment with fenfluramine and phentermine

☐ C Mitral stenosis occurs in association with the use of fenfluramine and phentermine

☐ D Selective serotonin re-uptake inhibitors cause heart valve abnormalities

☐ E Obesity *per se* is associated with a high prevalence of heart valve regurgitation

1.39 A 46-year-old man presents to the Emergency Department with a painful erection which is diagnosed as priapism. The attending physician feels that it is due to a drug that was started three weeks previously. Which one of the following drugs is associated with priapism?

☐ A Trazodone

☐ B Imipramine

☐ C Captopril

☐ D Atenolol

☐ E Digoxin

1.40 A six-year-old boy presents with an unintentional overdose of iron tablets. He is treated with antidotal therapy. Which one of the following is known to be an antidote for iron?

☐ Vitamin C

☐ Activated charcoal

☐ Desferrioxamine

☐ Fomepizole

☐ Dicobalt edetate

1.41   Which one of the following actions is mediated by the α-adrenoceptor?

☐ A   Bronchiolar constriction

☐ B   Decrease in gut motility

☐ C   Dilation of the splanchnic circulation

☐ D   Penile erection

☐ E   Relaxation of the pregnant uterus

1.42   Zanamivir in the treatment of influenza is characterised by all of the following, except:

☐ A   A bioavailability of less than 20%

☐ B   A decrease in bronchial air flow

☐ C   Increased release of virus from cells

☐ D   Reduced penetration of the virus into the respiratory mucosa

☐ E   Reduced severity of the illness

1.43   Cephalosporins:

☐ A   Can be used in the treatment of *Clostridium difficile* diarrhoea

☐ B   Can cause neutropenia and thrombocytopenia

☐ C   Do not have a β-lactam ring in their structure

☐ D   Have a 90% chance of causing allergy if the patient has had a previous reaction to penicillin

☐ E   In general have half-lives greater than ten hours

1.44   Which one of the following causes of hypercalcaemia is most likely to respond to treatment with corticosteroids?

☐ A   Milk-alkali syndrome

☐ B   Paget's disease

☐ C   Primary hyperparathyroidism

☐ D   Sarcoidosis

☐ E   Small-cell lung cancer

1.45   In relation to morphine, which one of the following statements is true?

- ☐ A   Approximately 8% of the population cannot convert codeine to morphine
- ☐ B   Morphine is more water-soluble than diamorphine
- ☐ C   Normal-release morphine has an onset of action within five minutes
- ☐ D   Peak drug levels after once-daily preparations of morphine are reached after 12 hours
- ☐ E   Pupillary constriction is an effect that is subject to tolerance

1.46   Regarding β-adrenoceptor antagonists:

- ☐ A   Atenolol is a cardiospecific drug
- ☐ B   Celiprolol increases total peripheral resistance
- ☐ C   Drugs with intrinsic sympathomimetic activity are less likely to cause bradycardia
- ☐ D   Esmolol is a long-acting drug used to treat patients with atrial arrhythmias
- ☐ E   Propranolol causes prolongation of the QT interval

1.47   Which one of the following is a known effect of the anticonvulsant phenytoin?

- ☐ A   Can cause selective IgA deficiency
- ☐ B   Causes arrhythmias in 10% of patients
- ☐ C   Displays first-order kinetics
- ☐ D   Efficacy in myoclonic epilepsy
- ☐ E   Osteoporosis is a known adverse effect

1.48   The following are well-known drug-drug interactions. Which one of these can be considered to be a beneficial interaction and has been used therapeutically?

- ☐ A   Cimetidine and dapsone
- ☐ B   Cimetidine and phenytoin
- ☐ C   Cisapride and erythromycin
- ☐ D   Rifampicin and ciclosporin A
- ☐ E   Ritonavir and fluoxetine

1.49   Severe poisoning with iron is characterised by which one of the following?

☐ A   Blood glucose > 8.3 mmol/l

☐ B   Hypertension

☐ C   Normal plain abdominal X-ray

☐ D   Pulmonary haemorrhage

☐ E   Total white cell count of < 4 x 10^9/l

1.50   Which one of the following statements relating to the use of acetylcholinesterase inhibitors in the treatment of Alzheimer's disease is true?

☐ B   Donepezil binds to the esteratic site of the enzyme

☐ E   Donepezil has a half-life of seven hours

☐ A   Metrifonate binds reversibly to the active site of the enzyme

☐ C   Rivastigmine binds to both the anionic and esteratic sites of the enzyme

☐ D   The metabolite of metrifonate does not possess any pharmacological activity

1.51   Below is a list of drugs with their putative adverse reactions. Which one of the pairings is not correct?

☐ A   Cerivastatin – rhabdomyolysis

☐ B   Indinavir – renal stones

☐ C   Pergolide – pulmonary fibrosis

☐ D   Tolcapone – neuroleptic malignant syndrome

☐ E   Vigabatrin – anterior uveitis

1.52   Which one of the following statements about leflunomide is incorrect?

☐ A   It can be classed as a disease-modifying antirheumatic drug

☐ B   It has active metabolites

☐ C   It has comparable efficacy to sulfasalazine and methotrexate

☐ D   It inhibits dihydro-orotate dehydrogenase

☐ E   It inhibits purine synthesis

1.53 **During warfarin therapy which one of the following statements is correct?**

   ☐ A   Dosage is adjusted by monitoring drug levels

   ☐ B   Dose requirements are genetically determined

   ☐ C   Osteoporosis may develop

   ☐ D   Overdose can be reversed by protamine sulphate

   ☐ E   Therapeutic effect is usually achieved within 24 hours

1.54 **When inducing local anaesthesia by infiltration, which one of the following is correct?**

   ☐ A   Accidental injection of lidocaine (lignocaine) into the systemic circulation may increase myocardial and neuronal excitability

   ☐ B   Bupivacaine produces a shorter-lasting anaesthesia than lidocaine

   ☐ C   The anaesthetic agents used are strongly acidic

   ☐ D   The duration of anaesthesia may be prolonged by the addition of salbutamol

   ☐ E   The duration of anaesthesia with lidocaine depends on diffusion and not on drug metabolism

1.55 **Which one of the following statements regarding combined hormonal oral contraceptives is incorrect?**

   ☐ A   Oestrogen preparations promote blood clotting

   ☐ B   Oestrogens inhibit follicle stimulating hormone (FSH) release

   ☐ C   Progestogens inhibit luteinising hormone (LH) release

   ☐ D   The incidence of benign breast disease may be increased

   ☐ E   The risk of stroke is increased to a small extent

1.56 **In relation to the use of interferon-β in the treatment of multiple sclerosis, which one of the following is incorrect?**

   ☐ A   Does not have a beneficial effect if administered at the time of the first-ever demyelinating event

   ☐ B   Reduces brain atrophy

   ☐ C   Reduces relapses in patients with chronic multiple sclerosis

   ☐ D   Reduces the development of brain lesions on magnetic resonance imaging (MRI)

   ☐ E   Slows progression of physical disability

1.57 **Which one of the following antidepressants is least likely to cause anticholinergic side-effects?**

- ☐ A Amitriptyline
- ☐ B Clomipramine
- ☐ C Dothiepin
- ☐ D Lofepramine
- ☐ E Trazodone

1.58 **Concerning sumatriptan:**

- ☐ A Bioavailability after oral and subcutaneous administration is equivalent
- ☐ B It can be used safely in patients with known coronary artery disease
- ☐ C It can be used together with ergotamine in migraine
- ☐ D It inhibits the release of calcitonin gene-related peptide (CGRP)
- ☐ E It prevents the aura associated with migraine

1.59 **Concerning bupropion:**

- ☐ A It can cause Stevens–Johnson syndrome
- ☐ B It is a selective inhibitor of the neuronal uptake of noradrenaline (norepinephrine)
- ☐ C It is an enzyme inhibitor
- ☐ D It is effective in smoking cessation
- ☐ E It should not be used in patients with a history of seizures

1.60 **Which one of the following CNS-active drugs should be avoided in breast-feeding mothers?**

- ☐ A Codeine
- ☐ B Hyoscine
- ☐ C Neostigmine
- ☐ D Oxcarbazepine
- ☐ E Propranolol

1.61 **Which one of the following drugs is not used to treat minimal-change glomerulonephritis?**

☐ A   Chlorambucil

☐ B   Cyclophosphamide

☐ C   Ciclosporin

☐ D   Prednisolone

☐ E   Vincristine

1.62 **In relation to analgesic nephropathy, which one of the following statements is correct?**

☐ A   Analgesic nephropathy was previously the commonest cause of renal failure in Australia

☐ B   Onset of analgesic nephropathy is common after a week of heavy analgesic use

☐ C   Phenacetin has not been implicated in the aetiology of analgesic nephropathy

☐ D   Renal transplantation is contraindicated in cases of analgesic nephropathy

☐ E   The renal lesion in analgesic nephropathy is unique

1.63 **Which one of the following statements is not correct in relation to the nephrotoxicity of drugs?**

☐ A   Aminoglycosides cause proximal tubular necrosis

☐ B   Amphotericin B reduces renal blood flow

☐ C   Analgesic nephropathy is characterised pathologically by glomerulonephritis

☐ D   Gold is associated with glomerulonephritis

☐ E   Lithium carbonate causes nephrogenic diabetes insipidus

1.64 **With respect to therapeutic drug monitoring for a patient with renal failure, which one of the following statements is correct?**

☐ A   Concomitant administration of diuretics makes aminoglycoside toxicity more likely

☐ B   Steady-state levels of theophylline can be measured after two half-lives of the drug

☐ C   The only way to avoid toxicity is to reduce the dose of a potentially toxic drug

☐ D   Therapeutic concentrations of vancomycin are unlikely to be maintained beyond 24 hours after dosage

☐ E   When giving gentamicin, a trough level is sufficient to determine dosage adjustment

1.65 **Which one of the following drugs does not cause constipation?**

☐ A   Cholestyramine

☐ B   Disopyramide

☐ C   Nifedipine

☐ D   Tricyclic antidepressants (TCA)

☐ E   Verapamil

1.66 **A 67-year-old gentleman with a history of alcohol excess is admitted for the third time with a large haematemesis due to previously diagnosed oesophageal varices. Which one of the following therapies has been shown to reduce mortality in the acute situation?**

☐ A   Antibiotics

☐ B   Glypressin

☐ C   Intravenous ranitidine

☐ D   Octreotide

☐ E   Propranolol

1.67 **Which one of the following drugs can safely be used in liver failure without dose adjustment?**

☐ A Digoxin

☐ B Erythromycin

☐ C Metformin

☐ D Morphine

☐ E Propranolol

1.68 **When considering paracetamol overdose, which one of the following is least likely to increase the risk of liver damage occurring?**

☐ A Acute alcohol intake

☐ B Anorexia nervosa

☐ C Concomitant therapy with isoniazid

☐ D Concomitant therapy with phenytoin

☐ E HIV-positive status

1.69 **Methotrexate acts by:**

☐ A Binding to DNA

☐ B Increasing the metabolism of folic acid derivatives

☐ C Inhibition of dihydrofolate oxidase

☐ D Inhibiting DNA polymerase

☐ E Reducing nucleotide biosynthesis

1.70 **Lung fibrosis can be caused by:**

☐ A 5-Fluorouracil

☐ B Busulfan

☐ C Cyclophosphamide

☐ D Cytarabine

☐ E Vincristine

1.71 **During the cell cycle, 5-fluorouracil exerts its actions predominantly during:**

☐ A   Cell differentiation

☐ B   The G0 phase

☐ C   The G1 and S phases

☐ D   The G2 and M phases

☐ E   The S and G2 phases

1.72 **Hydroxyurea is commonly used in the treatment of which one of the following?**

☐ A   Acute lymphocytic leukaemia

☐ B   Breast carcinoma

☐ C   Carcinoma of the cervix

☐ D   Chronic myeloid leukaemia

☐ E   Non-Hodgkin's lymphoma

1.73 **In patients with suspected acute intermittent porphyria, which one of the following drugs should be avoided?**

☐ A   Amoxicillin

☐ B   Dapsone

☐ C   Gentamicin

☐ D   Griseofulvin

☐ E   Tetracycline

1.74 **Which one of the following may help reduce insulin resistance?**

☐ A   Acarbose

☐ B   Atenolol

☐ C   High-dose bendroflumethiazide (bendrofluazide)

☐ D   Metformin

☐ E   Prednisolone

1.75 **Which one of the following is true of the selective estrogen receptor modulator (SERM), raloxifene?**

- ☐ A   Associated with an increased risk of breast carcinoma
- ☐ B   Is extensively renally excreted
- ☐ C   Reduces the risk of non-vertebral body fractures
- ☐ D   Reduces the risk of vertebral fractures by 30%
- ☐ E   Results in vaginal bleeding

1.76 **In a hypertensive patient with diabetic nephropathy, which one of the following should be the drug of first choice?**

- ☐ A   Atenolol
- ☐ B   Bendroflumethiazide (bendrofluazide)
- ☐ C   Captopril
- ☐ D   Diltiazem
- ☐ E   Doxazosin

IMMUNOLOGY

Best of Five

Questions

For each of the questions select the ONE most appropriate answer from the options provided.

2.1 A 23-year-old man is admitted with a short history of myalgia and a papular, purpuric rash on his legs. Investigations show: normal full blood count, including platelet count, alanine aminotranferase (ALT) mildly elevated at 67 U/l (normal range 5–45 U/l) and other liver function tests are normal. Dipstick urinalysis shows blood ++, protein ++. Antinuclear antibodies (ANA) and antibodies to neutrophil cytoplasm (ANCA) negative, rheumatoid factor positive at 1/256 (normal < 1/32), complement C3 1.2 g/l (normal range 0.6–1.6 g/l), complement C4 < 0.01 g/l (normal range 0.2–0.4 g/l). Which one of the following is the most likely diagnosis?

☐ A Hereditary angio-oedema

☐ B Henoch–Schönlein purpura

☐ C Mixed cryoglobulinaemia

☐ D Systemic lupus erythematosus

☐ E Rheumatoid arthritis

2.2 A 27-year-old man is admitted with a hot and swollen left knee. He has a history of recurrent chest infections. Culture of aspirated synovial fluid shows a pure growth of *Streptococcus pneumoniae*. Further investigation reveals that his serum immunoglobulins are reduced: IgG 0.8 g/l (normal range 6.5–16 g/l), IgA 0.1 g/l (normal range 0.6–5 g/l), IgM 0.2 g/l (normal range 0.6–3.2 g/l). Which one of the following is the most likely underlying diagnosis?

☐ A HIV infection

☐ B Primary antibody deficiency

☐ C Coeliac disease

☐ D Multiple myeloma

☐ E Cystic fibrosis

2.3   An 18-year-old man presents with a history of chronic ill health and
       recurrent infection. At the age of four he was treated for pneumonia and at
       the age of seven he had a prolonged admission with staphylococcal
       osteomyelitis of the right tibia. He reports that his brother died aged six from
       'fungal pneumonia'. He now has fever, a persistent productive cough and a
       chest X-ray reveals a cavitating lesion in the right mid-zone. Microscopy of
       his sputum shows hyphae suggestive of *Aspergillus*. Which one of the
       following investigations is most likely to point to the underlying diagnosis?

☐ A   Serum immunoglobulins

☐ B   Neutrophil function tests

☐ C   CD4 count

☐ D   Karyotyping

☐ E   Tests for ciliary dysfunction

2.4   A 23-year-old woman collapses at a party after eating some chocolate. She
       develops an urticarial rash, marked bronchospasm and on assessment by
       the paramedics her blood pressure is 70/50 mmHg. After treatment she
       gives a history of peanut allergy. What pathological mechanism is most
       likely to have immediately precipitated her collapse?

☐ A   Development of a TH2 response against peanut antigens

☐ B   A genetic predisposition to produce high levels of IgE

☐ C   Cross-linking of antigen-specific IgE bound to high-affinity IgE receptors

☐ D   Release of mast cell tryptase

☐ E   Activation of the sympathetic nervous system

2.5   A 24-year-old woman presents with diabetic ketoacidosis. She is treated
       and stabilised on insulin. Two years later she presents with lethargy and
       cold intolerance and is found to be myxoedematous. At the age of 30 she
       presents with marked fatigue and myalgia. Control of her diabetes and
       thyroid function have always been impeccable and her Hb A_{1c} is 5.4%.
       Which one of the following disorders is most likely to be the cause of her
       symptoms?

☐ A   Myasthenia gravis

☐ B   Primary ovarian failure

☐ C   Coeliac disease

☐ D   Addison's disease

☐ E   Pernicious anaemia

2.6   **T cells commonly secrete which one of the following cytokines when stimulated?**

☐   A   IL-1 and tumour necrosis factor-β (TNF-β)

☐   B   Interferon-β (IFN-β)

☐   C   Interleukin-1 (IL-1) and interferon-β (IFN-β)

☐   D   Interleukin-2 (IL-2) and interferon-γ (IFN-γ)

☐   E   Tumour necrosis factor-α (TNF-α)

2.7   **In autoimmunity, which one of the following pairings correctly matches cell type with site of immune surveillance?**

☐   A   All of the options

☐   B   B cell/bone marrow

☐   C   B cell/thymus

☐   D   T cell/bone marrow

☐   E   T cell/spleen

2.8   **Which one of the following immunodeficiency disorders is not associated with a primary B-cell abnormality?**

☐   A   Common variable immunodeficiency

☐   B   DiGeorge syndrome

☐   C   IgA deficiency

☐   D   Wiskott–Aldrich syndrome

☐   E   X-linked (Bruton's) agammaglobulinaemia

2.9   **Type II cryoglobulinaemia is most often associated with which one of these conditions?**

☐   A   Hepatitis C

☐   B   Multiple myeloma

☐   C   Rheumatoid arthritis

☐   D   Systemic lupus eythematosus

☐   E   Waldenström's macroglobulinaemia

2.10 **A Fab fragment of an immunoglobulin constitutes which one of the following?**

☐ A The Fab portion of one heavy chain linked to one light chain

☐ B The hypervariable region of the light and heavy chains

☐ C The variable region of the light chain

☐ D The variable region of the heavy chain

☐ E Two Fab portions of one heavy chain linked to two light chains

INFECTIOUS DISEASES

Best of Five

Questions

INFECTIOUS DISEASES: 'BEST OF FIVE' QUESTIONS

For each of the questions select the ONE most appropriate answer from the options provided.

3.1 **Which one of the following molecules is the target for a licensed HIV drug treatment?**

☐ A CD4

☐ B gp41

☐ C CCR5

☐ D CXCR4

☐ E p24

3.2 **Which one of the following statements about the prion protein is true?**

☐ A Prion protein is encoded on the host genome

☐ B The amino acid sequence of the prion protein in variant Creutzfeldt–Jakob disease (vCJD) is the same as that in bovine spongiform encephalopathy

☐ C The risk of early or late onset of disease cannot be predicted

☐ D The infectivity of prion protein can be reduced by nucleases

☐ E Tonsillar biopsy can assist in the diagnosis of sporadic Creutzfeldt–Jakob disease

3.3 **A patient with HIV has a CD4 count of 25×10^6 cells/l. It is likely that he will respond poorly to any vaccination, but which vaccine is absolutely contraindicated?**

☐ A Hepatitis B vaccine

☐ B Hepatitis A vaccine

☐ C Pneumococcal vaccine

☐ D Yellow fever vaccine

☐ E Rabies vaccine

3.4 In the UK there is a legal duty on the attending physician to notify a number of infectious diseases to the Consultant in Communicable Disease Control. Other infections should be reported as a matter of good practice if there is a public health implication. Which one of the following infections is a legally notifiable disease?

☐ A Brucellosis

☐ B Q fever

☐ C Legionnaires' disease

☐ D Lyme disease

☐ E Hepatitis C

3.5 A 25-year-old Australian backpacker swam in Lake Malawi four months ago. He now has a peripheral blood eosinophilia and bloody diarrhoea. Which one of the following investigations is most likely to confirm the diagnosis?

☐ A Stool culture

☐ B Midnight blood sample for the presence of microfilaria

☐ C Amoebic serology

☐ D Rectal biopsy

☐ E Thick blood film for trypanosomes

3.6 A 50-year-old UK-born man has been on a walking safari in a game park in northern South Africa, never having previously been out of Europe. He presents seven days later with a fever and two black scabbing lesions on his legs. Two other people in his party of 20 also have a similar illness. What is the most appropriate treatment?

☐ A Co-amoxiclav

☐ B Doxycycline

☐ C Praziquantel

☐ D Sodium stibogluconate

☐ E Melarsoprol

3.7   A 30-year-old UK man who has had a regular sexual partner and no other partners over the previous two years presents with a urethral discharge and discomfort on passing urine. Clinical examination is unremarkable. Moderately abundant neutrophil polymorphs, but no organisms, are seen on the Gram stain of the urethral discharge. Which is the most likely causative organism?

    ☐ A   *Treponema pallidum*

    ☐ B   *Chlamydia trachomatis*

    ☐ C   *Trichomonas vaginalis*

    ☐ D   Herpes simplex

    ☐ E   *Neisseria gonorrhoeae*

3.8   A 20-year-old man arrives in the UK with a mosquito-borne illness. He is transferred to a specialist unit. The referral letter states that he has just arrived in the UK from India but you know that this travel history must be wrong. Which infection does he have?

    ☐ A   *Wuchereria bancrofti* filariasis

    ☐ B   Japanese encephalitis

    ☐ C   Dengue fever

    ☐ D   Yellow fever

    ☐ E   *Plasmodium vivax* malaria

3.9   A 17-year-old boy develops a sore throat with enlarged tonsils and generalised lymphadenopathy. A blood film shows an excess of atypical lymphocytes and a Paul–Bunnell test is strongly positive. Which one of the following is true?

    ☐ A   The sore throat should be treated with co-amoxiclav

    ☐ B   The atypical lymphocytes are activated B lymphocytes

    ☐ C   The Paul–Bunnell test detects neutralising antibodies directed against Epstein–Barr virus

    ☐ D   Tonsillar enlargement causing respiratory obstruction should be treated with ganciclovir

    ☐ E   Persistent, uncontrolled infection can occur as an X-linked condition in males

3.10 An established surgeon in the UK who was hepatitis B surface antigen-negative seven years ago is now found to be hepatitis B surface antigen-positive. Which one of the following statements is most likely to be true?

- ❏ A The diagnosis must be wrong as she is known to have been vaccinated against hepatitis B

- ❏ B Treatment with a nucleoside reverse transcriptase inhibitor may be indicated

- ❏ C She can continue to work if the hepatitis B e antigen is negative

- ❏ D She must have contracted hepatitis B from an unnoticed needlestick injury from a patient

- ❏ E Patients she has operated on in the past six weeks should be offered hepatitis B immunoglobulin

3.11 A 54-year-old woman born in the Midwest USA and resident in the UK for the past 15 years (with her most recent visit back to the Midwest USA six months ago) develops an acute pneumonia. Two sets of blood cultures taken prior to the start of antibiotic treatment are negative. Which one of the following statements is most likely to be correct?

- ❏ A The causative agent is unlikely to be *Streptococcus pneumoniae*

- ❏ B Negative *Coxiella burnetii* serology taken on day 3 of the illness effectively excludes Q fever

- ❏ C Negative *Legionella* urinary antigen effectively excludes *Legionella*

- ❏ D The illness is highly unlikely to be acute pulmonary histoplasmosis

- ❏ E The presence of cold agglutinins is suggestive of *Mycoplasma* infection but it is a highly non-specific test

3.12 A herdsman from the Middle East is admitted with a three-day history of fever shortly after his arrival in the UK. A zoonosis is suspected. His white blood cell count and platelet count are normal, but his C-reactive protein is elevated. A thick blood film stained with Giemsa stain does not show any parasites. Blood cultures become positive after five days' incubation. Which of the following is the most likely disease?

- ❏ A Brucellosis

- ❏ B Rift Valley fever (RVF)

- ❏ C Q fever

- ❏ D Sleeping sickness

- ❏ E Crimea Congo haemorrhagic fever (CCHF)

3.13   A patient with advanced AIDS, who has never travelled outside the UK, develops severe *Pneumocystis jiroveci* pneumonia and requires ventilation on the Intensive Care Unit. Blood cultures taken on days 10, 11 and 12 of the ICU stay all grow a fungus. Which is the most likely organism?

❏   A   *Candida albicans*

❏   B   *Aspergillus fumigatus*

❏   C   *Pneumocystis jiroveci*

❏   D   *Histoplasma capsulatum*

❏   E   *Coccidioides immitis*

3.14   A previously fit 25-year-old man develops mild nausea two weeks into a course of treatment for smear-positive pulmonary tuberculosis. He has been prescribed correct doses of rifampicin, isoniazid, ethambutol and pyrazinamide. Full blood count, urea and electrolytes are normal. Alkaline phosphatase and serum bilirubin are normal. Alanine aminotransferase (ALT) is 153 U/l and aspartate transaminase (AST) is 160 U/l. A clotting screen is normal. What is the most appropriate course of action?

❏   A   Immediately stop all treatment and repeat liver function tests in one week, re-introducing treatment gradually when liver function tests are normal

❏   B   Add pyridoxine to medication

❏   C   Temporarily stop rifampicin, isoniazid and pyrazinamide, continuing the ethambutol

❏   D   Continue all medication and repeat liver function tests in one week

❏   E   Reduce the doses of rifampicin, isoniazid and pyrazinamide

3.15   A 30-year-old woman from sub-Saharan Africa is diagnosed with advanced
       HIV (CD4 count 30 × 10⁶/l) and cervical lymph node and pulmonary
       tuberculosis. She is commenced on prophylactic co-trimoxazole,
       combination antiretroviral therapy and a standard quadruple
       antituberculous therapy (with doses adjusted correctly to compensate for
       drug interactions). Four weeks later she develops enlargement of her
       cervical lymph nodes, which ulcerate and discharge, shortness of breath
       and worsening of the pulmonary infiltrates on chest X-ray. What is the most
       likely explanation?

   ❑   A   Drug-resistant tuberculosis
   ❑   B   Superadded infection with another opportunistic agent
   ❑   C   Development of non-Hodgkin's lymphoma
   ❑   D   Enhanced antimycobacterial immune reaction
   ❑   E   Drug reaction

3.16   A 35-year-old HIV-positive man has been taking zidovudine, lamivudine
       and nevirapine for the past two years, during which time he has been
       extremely well, with a CD4 count between 500 and 600 × 10⁶/l and HIV
       viral load less than 50 copies/ml. However his most recent blood test
       shows that his CD4 count has fallen to 150 × 10⁶/l and his HIV viral load
       has risen to 400,000 copies/ml. He comes to the clinic for the results of his
       blood tests. Which one of the following would you do at this clinic visit?

   ❑   A   Request sequencing of his HIV to look for mutations indicating
            resistance to antiretroviral drugs
   ❑   B   Add in a new antiretroviral agent that he has not had before
   ❑   C   Measure serum p24 antigen
   ❑   D   Change all his antiretroviral medication to a new combination
   ❑   E   Start prophylaxis against *Mycobacterium avium-intracellulare* (MAI)

3.17   A 40-year-old woman, recently arrived in the UK from southern Sudan, presents with a two-month history of fever, marked hepatosplenomegaly and general wasting. Blood tests show her to be anaemic with a low platelet count, low albumin and high IgG. Repeated thin malaria films are negative. What would be the next investigation of choice?

❑   A   Slit skin smear

❑   B   Bone marrow aspirate

❑   C   Thick blood film

❑   D   Liver biopsy

❑   E   Mantoux test

3.18   A 20-year-old leukaemic patient from the Middle East who has had a bone marrow transplant six weeks ago develops an anaemia which responds to intravenous immunoglobulin. Which infectious agent is the likely cause?

❑   A   Parvovirus B19

❑   B   Cytomegalovirus

❑   C   Adenovirus

❑   D   *Mycobacterium tuberculosis*

❑   E   *Aspergillus fumigatus*

3.19   A 53-year-old man recently arrived from Ghana is diagnosed with *Plasmodium falciparum* malaria. A blood film shows that 40% of his red blood cells contain malaria parasites. His renal function is impaired and his conscious level is deteriorating. In addition to immediate resuscitation, which of the following is the first measure you would institute?

❑   A   Atovaquone/proguanil combination therapy

❑   B   Quinine

❑   C   Chloroquine

❑   D   Haemofiltration

❑   E   Exchange transfusion

3.20   A 50-year-old man presents with a fever five days following his return from an eight-week holiday in Thailand. He is jaundiced but has no evidence of liver failure. He has marked renal impairment. He has a diminished cardiac output and an echocardiogram is consistent with a myocarditis. He subsequently develops pulmonary haemorrhage. What is the most likely diagnosis?

- ❑ A   Scrub typhus (*Orientia tsutsugamushi*)
- ❑ B   Leptospirosis
- ❑ C   Typhoid fever
- ❑ D   Melioidosis (*Burkholderia pseudomallei*)
- ❑ E   Severe falciparum malaria

3.21   A 23-year-old man is investigated for hepatitis B virus (HBV) infection. Positive tests are found for hepatitis B surface antigen (HBsAg) and IgM antibodies to the core antigen (anti-HBc IgM) and a negative 'e' antigen (eAg). Which one of the following is the most likely clinical status?

- ❑ A   Acute HBV infection
- ❑ B   Chronic HBV carrier
- ❑ C   Convalescence from acute HBV
- ❑ D   None of the options
- ❑ E   Previous immunisation against HBV

3.22   Which one of the following viral groups is least associated with haemorrhagic manifestations?

- ❑ A   Arbovirus
- ❑ B   Arenavirus
- ❑ C   Paramyxovirus
- ❑ D   Picornavirus
- ❑ E   Rotavirus

3.23   When comparing Rhodesian and Gambian sleeping sickness, which one of the following statements is not true of both conditions?

- ❑ A   CNS abnormalities occur
- ❑ B   Hepatosplenomegaly occurs
- ❑ C   Humans are a recognised reservoir
- ❑ D   Melarsoprol is effective treatment
- ❑ E   The causative agent is *Trypanosoma brucei*

3.24 **In which one of the following malarial agents does a stage of exoerythrocytic schizogony definitely not occur?**

❏ E   None of the options

❏ C   *Plasmodium falciparum*

❏ B   *Plasmodium malariae*

❏ D   *Plasmodium ovale*

❏ A   *Plasmodium vivax*

3.25 **A 43-year-old male African immigrant, recently arrived in the UK, is assessed by his general practitioner during registration. He has a long-standing right hemiplegia and is blind in his left eye. There is a history of recurrent pain and redness of the eyes with an occasional exudative discharge. The general practitioner notes several small hard subcutaneous nodules. Which one of the following is the most likely diagnosis?**

❏ A   Cysticercosis

❏ B   Filariasis

❏ C   Hydatid disease

❏ D   Schistosomiasis

❏ E   Strongyloidiasis

3.26 **All the following statements regarding Q fever are correct except which one?**

❏ A   Acute illness may resolve spontaneously without treatment

❏ B   Osteomyelitis is a recognised complication

❏ C   The causative agent is *Coxiella burnetii*

❏ D   The Weil–Felix reaction is positive

❏ E   Transmission of the disease to humans is independent of an arthropod vector

3.27 **Which one of the following is a high risk factor for contracting *Haemophilus*?**

❏ A   Alcohol abuse

❏ B   All of the options

❏ C   Infancy and early childhood

❏ D   Sickle cell disease

❏ E   Splenectomy

3.28   A 40-year-old British abattoir worker becomes systemically ill with jaundice, microscopic haematuria and meningism. He is found to have mild renal impairment, and haemolytic anaemia. There is no rash, pharyngitis or lymphadenopathy. He has not travelled abroad. Which one of the following is the most probable diagnosis?

     ❑   A   Cholera

     ❑   B   Coxsackievirus A

     ❑   C   Infectious mononucleosis

     ❑   D   Leptospirosis

     ❑   E   Sporotrichosis

3.29   Which one of the following statements regarding staphylococcal and streptococcal infection is incorrect?

     ❑   A   Bacteraemia is uncommon in toxic shock syndrome

     ❑   B   Group A *Streptococcus* causes erysipelas

     ❑   C   Impetigo is associated with glomerulonephritis

     ❑   D   None of the options

     ❑   E   Scalded skin syndrome is caused by *Staphylococcus aureus*

3.30   A leukaemic patient on chemotherapy presents with fever and a pulmonary infiltrate. Which one of the following infectious agents could present in this way?

     ❑   A   All of the options

     ❑   B   *Chlamydia*

     ❑   C   *Cryptococcus*

     ❑   D   Herpes simplex

     ❑   E   None of the options

3.31 A 26-year-old man with a history of injecting drugs is admitted with fever and malaise. His temperature is 39.3 °C, pulse 126 bpm and blood pressure 90/65 mmHg. He is mildly confused, but without symptoms of meningism or focal neurological signs. A loud murmur that increases with inspiration is audible at the lower left sternal edge. A plain chest X-ray shows several small cavitating lesions peripherally, but is otherwise normal. Which one of the following is the most likely diagnosis?

❏ A Acute HIV seroconversion illness

❏ B *Cryptococcus neoformans* infection

❏ C *Mycobacterium tuberculosis* infection

❏ D *Staphylococcus aureus* endocarditis and septicaemia

❏ E Tricuspid endocarditis due to *Streptococcus bovis*

3.32 Antibiotic chemotherapies employ several mechanisms of action. Some interfere with bacterial cell-wall synthesis and others penetrate well into cells and disrupt bacterial ribosomal function. Which one of the following drugs acts by interfering with ribosomal function?

❏ A Amoxicillin

❏ B Ciprofloxacin

❏ C Clarithromycin

❏ D Trimethoprim

❏ E Vancomycin

3.33 An 85-year-old Caucasian lady presents with fever, headache, neck stiffness and photophobia. She recently completed a three-day course of cefalexin for a urinary tract infection. Her past medical history is otherwise unremarkable. A lumbar puncture is performed and the cerebrospinal fluid (CSF) is found to be clear and colourless. The CSF biochemistry and microscopy shows a protein of 1.7 g/l, a glucose of 3.1 mmol/l (plasma glucose 6.8 mmol/l), and a white cell count of 104 per mm^3 (lymphocytes 65%, polymorphs 35%). Occasional short Gram-positive rods are present. Which one of the following is the likely cause of her meningitis?

❏ A *Listeria monocytogenes*

❏ B *Mycobacterium tuberculosis*

❏ C *Neisseria meningitidis*

❏ D *Pseudomonas aeruginosa*

❏ E *Streptococcus pneumoniae*

3.34 Cytomegalovirus (CMV) is an important opportunistic infection in immunocompromised individuals. Of the five clinical complications of HIV-infection listed below, which one would be least likely to be due to CMV infection?

- ❑ A   Acalculous cholecystitis
- ❑ B   Encephalitis
- ❑ C   Nephritis
- ❑ D   Polyradiculopathy
- ❑ E   Retinitis

3.35 Which one of the following is a chemokine co-receptor that acts in conjunction with the CD4+ receptor to enable attachment of the HIV virus, membrane fusion, and internalisation of the contents of the HIV virus into the host cytoplasm?

- ❑ A   CCR5
- ❑ B   CD8+
- ❑ C   gp120
- ❑ D   HIV protease enzyme
- ❑ E   Pol gene product

3.36 A 35-year-old man presents with a two-day history of fever, malaise, wheeze, mild diarrhoea, an urticarial rash and hepatosplenomegaly. He recently returned from a three-month overland trip in East Africa. He can recall numerous insect bites on his trip and his adherence to antimalarial prophylaxis has been poor. He swam in freshwater rivers and consumed local food and beverages. His full blood count on admission shows a normal haemoglobin and platelet count, but a raised white cell count of $15.7 \times 10^9/l$ (neutrophils 26%, lymphocytes 21%, eosinophils 45%, monocytes 1%). No malaria parasites are detected on three separate films. Which one of the following is the most likely diagnosis?

- ❑ A   Amoebiasis
- ❑ B   Dengue fever
- ❑ C   Leishmaniasis
- ❑ D   Malaria
- ❑ E   Schistosomiasis

3.37 A 43-year-old man, HIV-positive for ten years, stopped all antiretroviral treatments six months ago because of side-effects. His current CD4+ count is very low. Over the course of two months he has developed a hemiparesis and dysarthria, but has not been systemically unwell or febrile. A magnetic resonance imaging (MRI) scan of the brain shows multiple cerebral white matter lesions that do not enhance with contrast or show mass effect. Cerebro-spinal fluid examination is within normal limits. Which one of the following organisms is most likely to be responsible for his symptoms?

- ❏ A *Cryptococcus neoformans*
- ❏ B JC virus
- ❏ C *Mycobacterium tuberculosis*
- ❏ D *Nocardia asteroides*
- ❏ E *Toxoplasma gondii*

3.38 A 25-year-old woman is admitted to hospital acutely unwell with malaise, fever, profuse vomiting, and mild diarrhoea over a 36-hour period. There is no history of foreign travel and her food history is unremarkable. On admission her pulse is 130 bpm, blood pressure 84/62 mmHg, temperature 38.9 °C. She is confused, but has no focal neurology. She has a faint, erythematous rash, particularly noticeable on her extremities. Her tongue and buccal mucosa are noted to be red and hyperaemic. What is the most likely diagnosis?

- ❏ A *Escherichia coli* O157 infection
- ❏ B Meningococcal septicaemia
- ❏ C *Salmonella* gastroenteritis
- ❏ D Toxic shock syndrome
- ❏ E Typhoid fever

3.39 A 25-year-old man presents to a sexually transmitted diseases (STD) clinic. He moved to the UK from West Africa four years ago. Five days ago he developed a cluster of ten small (1–2-mm), painful, punched-out ulcers on the penis. The inguinal lymph nodes are tender and slightly enlarged, but there is no evidence of suppuration. He has had unprotected sex with a new partner recently. Which one of the following is the most likely diagnosis?

- ❑ A Behçet's disease
- ❑ B Chancroid
- ❑ C Genital herpes
- ❑ D Lymphogranuloma venereum (LGV)
- ❑ E Syphilis

3.40 Which one of the following statements regarding antituberculous medication is incorrect?

- ❑ A Capreomycin is ototoxic
- ❑ B Macrolides may increase the risk of rifabutin-induced uveitis
- ❑ C Rifampicin causes an orange discoloration of the urine and secretions
- ❑ D Rifampicin is a potent liver enzyme inducer
- ❑ E Toxic side-effects of isoniazid are best reduced by the concomitant use of rifabutin

RHEUMATOLOGY

Best of Five

Questions

RHEUMATOLOGY: 'BEST OF FIVE' QUESTIONS

For each of the questions select the ONE most appropriate answer from the options provided.

4.1 An 82-year-old woman presents with non-specific joint pain. She is found to have raised levels of IgM rheumatoid factor (RF) at a titre of 1/64. What is the most appropriate interpretation?

- ☐ A The presence of rheumatoid factor confirms a diagnosis of rheumatoid arthritis
- ☐ B Carriage of DR4 rheumatoid arthritis-associated alleles is the best predictor of erosive outcome
- ☐ C The prevalence of rheumatoid factor in the elderly is approximately 7%
- ☐ D Raised levels of IgM rheumatoid factor suggests that the patient has had a recent infection
- ☐ E Persistence of rheumatoid factor at high titre is a risk factor for the development of rheumatoid arthritis

4.2 A 68-year-old woman is diagnosed with rheumatoid arthritis on the basis of symmetrical polyarthritis, and the presence of rheumatoid nodules and erosions. She is prescribed a disease-modifying antirheumatic drug (DMARD). Which one of the following is not true?

- ☐ A Sulfasalazine is most likely to cause agranulocytosis soon after it is first taken
- ☐ B Worsening of rheumatoid nodules is a recognised complication of therapy with methotrexate
- ☐ C Hydroxychloroquine is associated with reversible corneal deposits
- ☐ D D-penicillamine is associated with drug-induced myasthaenia gravis
- ☐ E Hyperviscocity syndrome is a recognised complication of therapy with gold salts

4.3   **A 32-year-old man presents with a history of left-sided knee swelling following an episode of gastroenteritis. In the past he has had episodic low back pain. Which one of the following is the best response?**

- [ ] A   If he is found to carry the HLA-B27 antigen the course is more likely to be chronic
- [ ] B   Knee aspiration may reveal the presence of micro-organisms in the joint
- [ ] C   Absence of conjunctivitis excludes a diagnosis of reactive arthritis
- [ ] D   Sacro-iliitis is likely to be present on X-rays
- [ ] E   Antibiotics, if given at an early stage, can limit the extent of joint involvement

4.4   **A 56-year-old lady presents with joint pain, Raynaud's phenomenon and a photosensitive skin rash affecting her face, upper arms and neck. On examination, she is noted to have some proximal muscle weakness. ANA is positive and ribonucleoprotein (RNP) antibodies are negative. Which one of the following is the most likely diagnosis?**

- [ ] A   Systemic lupus erythematosus (SLE)
- [ ] B   Limited cutaneous systemic sclerosis
- [ ] C   Dermatomyositis
- [ ] D   Polymyositis
- [ ] E   Mixed connective tissue disease

4.5   **Which one of the following is not compatible with a diagnosis of Behçet's disease?**

- [ ] A   Chronic relapsing bilateral uveitis
- [ ] B   Amyloidosis associated with nephrotic syndrome
- [ ] C   Sacro-iliitis and oligoarthritis of the lower limbs
- [ ] D   Erythema nodosum
- [ ] E   Budd–Chiari syndrome

4.6   **A 54-year-old man presents with recurrent episodes of nasal swelling lasting approximately one week at a time. Which one of the following is not compatible with a diagnosis of relapsing polychondritis?**

- ☐ A   Diagnosis is confirmed on cartilage biopsy
- ☐ B   Recurrent episodes of ear swelling that spare the pinna
- ☐ C   A migratory non-erosive arthritis
- ☐ D   Response to treatment with colchicine
- ☐ E   Presence of bilateral iritis

4.7   **A 63-year-old man presents with a vasculitic skin rash, a peripheral neuropathy and gastrointestinal blood loss. He is found to have proteinuria on dipstick urinalysis. Which one of the following is the most likely diagnosis?**

- ☐ A   Microscopic polyangiitis
- ☐ B   Wegener's granulomatosus
- ☐ C   Henoch–Schönlein vasculitis
- ☐ D   Polyarteritis nodosa (PAN)
- ☐ E   Churg–Strauss syndrome

4.8   **A 72-year-old man complains of pain around the first metatarsophalangeal (MTP) joint of the left foot. He is otherwise well and is not on any medication. Which one of the following is the best response?**

- ☐ A   A raised uric acid level would confirm a diagnosis of gout
- ☐ B   Allopurinol should be commenced if episodes of joint pain are frequent
- ☐ C   Osteoarthritis is the most likely diagnosis
- ☐ D   A normal uric acid excludes a diagnosis of gout
- ☐ E   Presence of chondrocalcinosis would confirm a diagnosis of pseudogout

4.9   **A 65-year-old woman complains of difficulty lifting her arms above her head. Which one of the following is the most useful initial test to aid in diagnosis?**

- ☐ A   Muscle biopsy
- ☐ B   ESR
- ☐ C   Trial of steroids at 1 mg/kg/day
- ☐ D   Creatinine kinase
- ☐ E   Temporal artery biopsy

4.10 An 83-year-old lady with mobility problems is started on maintenance treatment with low-dose (7.5 mg/day) oral prednisolone for her rheumatoid arthritis. Which one of the following responses is the best?

- ☐ A Routine bone density scanning is not required as osteoprotection should be routinely prescribed in this situation
- ☐ B Etidronate should be added to her treatment
- ☐ C Routine calcium supplementation is unnecessary
- ☐ D When considering treatment decisions, results of bone density should be compared with an age-matched control
- ☐ E Osteoporosis is diagnosed when the T score is < -2.5

4.11 A 53-year-old lady complains of her fingers and toes turning white when she is working in the garden. On examination, she is noted to have sclerodactyly, oedema of her fingers and tight skin up to her upper arms. Which one of the following statements is the best response?

- ☐ A The diagnosis is limited cutaneous systemic sclerosis (CREST)
- ☐ B Treatment with penicillamine can reverse the skin changes
- ☐ C ACE inhibitors should be introduced as soon as any rise in blood pressure is noted
- ☐ D The most common cause of death is pulmonary hypertension
- ☐ E ANA may be positive

4.12 Which is the most common presentation of arthritis associated with sarcoidosis?

- ☐ A Self-limiting, benign condition principally affecting the lower limbs
- ☐ B Polyarthritis associated with bilateral hilar lymphadenopathy and erythema marginatum
- ☐ C Oligoarthritis affecting the lower limbs, associated with bilateral hilar lymphadenopathy and erythema nodosum
- ☐ D Polyarthritis associated with bilateral hilar lymphadenopathy and erythema nodosum
- ☐ E Asymmetrcal arthritis affecting the large joints of the upper limb and erythema chronicum migrans

4.13   A young man develops swelling of the distal interphalangeal (DIP) joints of the right middle and little and the left ring finger. He has had plaque psoriasis since the age of 28 and presents with nail pitting and onycholysis on examination. His IgM rheumatoid factor (RF) titre is positive at 1/32. Select the best response from the following statements:

  ☐ A   The presence of RF excludes a diagnosis of psoriatic arthritis

  ☐ B   Arthritis of the distal interphalangeal joints is usually associated with nail involvement

  ☐ C   Presence of HLA-B27 would confirm a diagnosis of psoriatic arthritis

  ☐ D   Chronic anterior uveitis is the characteristic ocular manifestation

  ☐ E   Antimalarials are contraindicated as they may exacerbate his skin psoriasis

4.14   **In septic arthritis, the commonest causative micro-organism is which one of the following?**

  ☐ A   *Streptococcus pyogenes*

  ☐ B   *Staphylococcus aureus*

  ☐ C   *Haemophilus influenzae*

  ☐ D   *Borrelia burgdorferi*

  ☐ E   *Neisseria gonorrhoeae*

4.15   **Which one of the following is the characteristic type of eye involvement in juvenile idiopathic arthritis?**

  ☐ A   Asymptomatic posterior uveitis

  ☐ B   Bilateral acute anterior uveitis

  ☐ C   Chronic anterior iridocyclitis

  ☐ D   Unilateral scleritis

  ☐ E   Bilateral conjunctivitis

4.16 A 50-year-old woman presents with knee pain. She is on medication for non-insulin-dependent diabetes mellitus, hypertension and moderate congestive cardiac failure. She has rheumatoid arthritis and is treated with methotrexate and low-dose prednisolone. She is commenced on a non-steroidal anti-inflammatory drug (NSAID). Which one of the following drugs can interact with the NSAID?

☐ A Angiotensin-converting enzyme (ACE) inhibitors

☐ B Any of these items

☐ C Methotrexate

☐ D Oral hypogylcaemics

☐ E Thiazide diuretics

4.17 A 72-year-old man presents to the Emergency Department with a low-trauma fracture to the wrist following a seizure. He has taken phenytoin for seizures, a β-blocker for hypertension, and prednisolone for polymyalgia rheumatica for many years. He complains of impotence and lethargy. In his history, which one of the following is not suggestive of a risk factor for osteoporosis?

☐ A Being male and 72 years of age

☐ B Impotence

☐ C Use of a β-blocker

☐ D Use of corticosteroids

☐ E Use of phenytoin

4.18 Which one of the following statements regarding drug-induced lupus (DIL) is not true?

☐ A Central nervous system and renal involvement is uncommon in DIL

☐ B Classical lupus skin findings (malar rash, oral ulcers, alopecia) are uncommon in DIL

☐ C Drugs implicated in the aetiology of DIL should not be used in idiopathic systemic lupus erythematosus

☐ D Methyldopa is implicated in causing DIL

☐ E More than 50% of patients taking procainamide for more than 12 months develop positive antinuclear antibody titres

4.19 Anti-neutrophil cytoplasmic antibodies (ANCA) are associated with which one of the following?

- ☐ A   All of the options
- ☐ B   Felty's syndrome
- ☐ C   Human immunodeficiency virus
- ☐ D   Inflammatory bowel disease
- ☐ E   Wegener's granulomatosis

4.20 A 24-year-old Iraqi man presents with recurrent attacks of generalised abdominal pain lasting up to 72 hours. He also describes a pleuritic-type pain, a swollen knee, and on more than one occasion has experienced a rash on his legs that is tender, swollen and well demarcated. Which one of the following statements is least likely to be true?

- ☐ A   A skin biopsy often demonstrates evidence of vasculitis
- ☐ B   Fever is often a reported complaint
- ☐ C   Persistent synovitis for more than a few months is uncommon
- ☐ D   Proteinuria may be present
- ☐ E   There is likely to be a leucocytosis

4.21 The following are all diagnostic criteria for benign joint hypermobility syndrome, except which one of the following?

- ☐ A   Back pain
- ☐ B   Beighton hypermobility score of 2 out of 9
- ☐ C   Herniae
- ☐ D   Joint pains in more than one joint for one week
- ☐ E   Soft tissue rheumatism in three or more sites

4.22 Which one of the following statements regarding uric acid metabolism is incorrect?

- ☐ A   None of the following
- ☐ B   Serum uric acid levels are increased in Fanconi's syndrome
- ☐ C   Serum uric acid levels increase in metabolic acidosis
- ☐ D   Spironolactone does not cause hyperuricaemia
- ☐ E   Toxaemia of pregnancy is associated with increased purine turnover

4.23 A 35-year-old woman is referred from her general practice following a presentation with shortness of breath, myalgia and arthralgia. Laboratory tests for extractable nuclear antigens are positive for anti-Sm, RNP, and Ro (SS-A). Which one of the following is the most likely diagnosis?

- [ ] A   Polymyositis
- [ ] B   Rheumatoid arthritis
- [ ] C   Sjögren's syndrome
- [ ] D   Systemic lupus erythematosus
- [ ] E   Systemic sclerosis

4.24 Which one of the following is a feature of aggressive disease in rheumatoid arthritis?

- [ ] A   All of the options
- [ ] B   Functional disability
- [ ] C   High rheumatoid factor titre
- [ ] D   Raised C-reactive protein
- [ ] E   Rheumatoid nodules

4.25 A 58-year-old man presents with blurred vision, an occipital headache, fatigue and shoulder girdle pain. On examination he has scalp tenderness, myalgia but no myopathy, and no evidence of fundoscopic or neurological abnormality. Which one of the following would be the correct immediate action?

- [ ] A   Commence a non-steroidal anti-inflammatory drug
- [ ] B   Commence oral prednisolone at 20 mg/day
- [ ] C   Request an ESR and temporal artery biopsy
- [ ] D   Request a computed tomography (CT) scan of the head
- [ ] E   Start the patient on 60 mg/day oral prednisolone

4.26   A 34-year-old hiker returned from a two-week vacation in the American Great Lakes four weeks ago. He complains of a flitting arthralgia, myalgia, bone pain and a swollen knee. He recalls an episode lasting several days on vacation where he had a headache, irritated eyes, a sore throat and swollen glands, and he has a persistent rash. He denies sexual contact. Which one of the following would be the most useful diagnostic test?

- [ ] A   Aspirate and culture the knee effusion for gonococcal infection
- [ ] B   Biopsy the rash or a palpable lymph node
- [ ] C   Measure serum antinuclear antibodies
- [ ] D   Measure spirochaete antibodies
- [ ] E   Measure the serum anti-streptolysin-O antibody titre (ASOT)

4.27   A 30-year-old woman collapses at her GP surgery. On arrival in the Emergency Department she is short of breath and hypoxic, with pleuritic-sounding chest pain. The patient is able to confirm that she is already on warfarin following a similar episode a year ago and that she lost a pregnancy in the first three months just two years ago. There is a family history of arthritis and her sister takes medication for a kidney disease. Which one of the following statements is least correct in this scenario?

- [ ] A   A dsDNA antibody titre could be useful
- [ ] B   Sudden widespread organ failure may occur
- [ ] C   There is a risk of arterial as well as venous thrombosis
- [ ] D   Thrombocytopenia may be present
- [ ] E   Warfarin should be dosed to maintain the INR at 2.0

4.28   Which one of the following is not a recognised cause of ectopic calcification or ossification of soft tissues?

- [ ] A   Dermatomyositis
- [ ] B   Hyperparathyroidism
- [ ] C   Hypothyroidism
- [ ] D   Trauma
- [ ] E   Tumour lysis

4.29 **Pyoderma gangrenosum is not a feature of which one of the following rheumatic diseases?**

- ☐ A   Churg–Strauss syndrome
- ☐ B   None of these
- ☐ C   Psoriatic arthritis
- ☐ D   Rheumatoid arthritis
- ☐ E   Wegener's granulomatosis

4.30 **A young man is diagnosed as having pseudohypoparathyroidism. Which one of the following laboratory tests is consistent with this diagnosis?**

- ☐ A   Low parathyroid levels
- ☐ B   Hypercalcaemia
- ☐ C   Hypophosphataemia
- ☐ D   None of these items
- ☐ E   Raised parathyroid hormone

CLINICAL PHARMACOLOGY: 'BEST OF FIVE' ANSWERS

1.1   A: Chloramphenicol

The mode of action of antibiotics can be classified as follows:

- Inhibition of bacterial cell wall synthesis: penicillins, cephalosporins, vancomycin and teicoplanin
- Inhibition of cell membrane synthesis: lincomycins
- Inhibition of protein synthesis: aminoglycosides, tetracycline, macrolides, chloramphenicol and clindamycin
- Inhibition of DNA synthesis: rifampicin, quinolone antibiotics, metronidazole, sulphonamides and trimethoprim.

1.2   A: Effective control of blood sugar has been shown to decrease long-term complications

In patients with IDDM, effective control of blood sugar has been shown to decrease long-term complications responsible for the morbidity and mortality of the disease. During an intercurrent infection, patients should not reduce insulin dosage as this may lead to diabetic ketoacidosis. Human insulin is now the most widely used form of insulin although some patients still use animal insulin. In theory, human insulin should be less immunogenic than porcine insulin, although this has not been borne out in clinical trials. Insulin lispro is an insulin analogue which is more rapidly absorbed; peak concentrations in blood occur earlier and loss from the circulation is more rapid. Insulin lispro therefore has a more rapid onset of action and post-prandial glucose concentrations do not rise as high as with soluble insulin and mild hypoglycaemia may be less common. Glycosylated haemoglobin (Hb A_{1C}) does not change very much with insulin lispro, possibly because blood glucose before the next meal tends to be higher than with soluble insulin.

1.3   C: It can cause retinopathy

Tamoxifen is a partial agonist of the oestrogen receptor. It behaves as an oestrogen antagonist in breast tissue but has weak agonist effects on the endometrium, bone remodelling and cholesterol metabolism. The drug's main use is in breast cancer where it is more effective in post-menopausal women than in pre-menopausal women. It is currently being tested to determine whether it prevents the development of breast cancer in women with a positive family history. Because of its partial agonist activity, it can lead to the development of endometrial cancer and of hypercalcaemia in patients with bony metastases. Tamoxifen also causes retinopathy, the mechanism of which is unclear. This is a relatively rare adverse effect, and does not require routine monitoring, but prescribers should be aware of its occurrence and should investigate for its presence when a patient complains of visual symptoms.

1.4   B: Insulin resistance

Protease inhibitors inhibit the viral aspartyl protease. They have largely been used in combination with two nucleoside analogues: such regimens have been shown to retard disease progression and decrease mortality. Protease inhibitors inhibit the cytochrome P450 enzymes and can therefore be responsible for clinically significant drug interactions with compounds such as midazolam (excess sedation) and rifabutin (uveitis). They have recently been reported to cause peripheral lipodystrophy which is characterised by fat redistribution, hypertension, hyperglycaemia, insulin resistance and possibly accelerated atherosclerosis. In light of this novel form of toxicity, their benefit-risk ratio needs to be re-evaluated.

1.5   B: Misoprostol

Warfarin, but not heparin, is associated with skeletal and CNS defects if the fetus is exposed in the first trimester, while exposure during the third trimester increases the risk of intracranial haemorrhage during delivery. Misoprostol is associated with the Moebius syndrome. Diazepam, oral contraceptives and aspirin were initially thought to possess some teratogenic risk but formal cohort and case-control studies and meta-analyses have provided some evidence that these drugs are safe.

1.6   B: It is associated with a twofold increased risk of breast cancer

Oestrogens should be combined with progestogens in patients with an intact uterus to reduce the risk of endometrial cancer, but can be used by themselves in patients who have had a hysterectomy. HRT has many benefits, including prevention of bone loss and possibly dementia, and the relief of menopausal symptoms. There are also many risks, including an increased risk of endometrial cancer (even in patients taking combined hormone therapy), breast cancer (approximately twofold) and venous thromboembolism. The beneficial effect of HRT on bone loss is more marked in patients who begin therapy within five years after the menopause. Raloxifene is a new non-steroidal selective oestrogen receptor modulator (SERM), which is just as effective as conventional forms of hormone replacement therapy. It has oestrogenic effects on bone and serum lipids, but does not stimulate endometrial growth (ie it exerts an anti-oestrogenic effect). Preliminary findings suggest that it is also protective against breast cancer.

1.7   C: Activated charcoal reduces the enterohepatic circulation of drugs

Gastric lavage is best reserved for patients who present within one hour of an overdose, although with drugs which reduce gastric emptying, such as, anticholinergics, the time interval can be longer. Ipecacuanha syrup is associated with an increased risk of aspiration pneumonitis and oesophageal damage and should not be used. Haemodialysis is useful for drugs with a low volume of distribution (ie drugs such as aspirin which reside mostly within the plasma) and is not used for drugs with a high volume of distribution, such as tricyclic antidepressants. Forced alkaline diuresis should only be considered in very severe cases of aspirin poisoning.

1.8   B: Ciclosporin

Grapefruit juice contains compounds which are inhibitors of the cytochrome P450 isoform CYP3A4. The ability of grapefruit juice to inhibit drug metabolism was first shown with the calcium-channel blocker felodipine. Subsequent investigations have shown that grapefruit juice can interact with many CYP3A4 substrates, including terfenadine (leading to QT prolongation), cisapride (QT prolongation), ciclosporin (ciclosporin toxicity), and the protease inhibitors. The interaction with the protease inhibitors can in fact be used therapeutically to increase their bioavailability and thus their effectiveness.

1.9   E: Genetically determined deficiencies of some of the drug metabolising enzymes have been described

Drug metabolism is conventionally divided into two phases – phase I and phase II. The main role of drug metabolism is to convert lipophilic compounds into hydrophilic metabolites which can then be excreted from the body. Drug metabolism can also result in the formation of toxic metabolites that may be responsible for idiosyncratic toxicity. In addition, it can result in the formation of active metabolites, such as norfluoxetine in the case of fluoxetine. Phase I pathways are usually catalysed by cytochrome P450 enzymes, of which there are many different isoforms, while phase II pathways are catalysed by a number of enzymes, including glucuronyl transferase and N-acetyltransferase. Many of these enzymes can be either inhibited or induced and some also show genetically determined deficiencies. For example, fluoxetine is metabolised by the P450 isoform CYP2D6, which is deficient in 6–10% of the UK population. Metabolism occurs in all organs, apart from those of ectodermal origin. The liver is the main site; other sites include skin, gut wall, kidney, lungs and brain.

1.10   A: Less likely to cause parkinsonism

Typical neuroleptic drugs such as chlorpromazine have been used for many years in the treatment of schizophrenia. Their usefulness is limited by their propensity to cause extrapyramidal adverse effects. Atypical neuroleptics are less likely to cause extrapyramidal adverse effects. In addition, they affect not only the positive symptoms (like the typical neuroleptics), but also affect the negative symptoms which are not improved by the typical neuroleptics. In comparison to the typical neuroleptics, the atypical neuroleptics are less likely to cause neuroleptic malignant syndrome and hyperprolactinaemia (except perhaps risperidone), but are more likely to induce weight gain. Atypical neuroleptics include clozapine, risperidone, olanzapine, sertindole, and quetiapine.

1.11   E: Inhibition of GABA transaminase

Anticonvulsants often have more than one mode of action, although their efficacy can often be rationalised on the basis of one main mode of action. In general, the mode of action of anticonvulsants can be divided into one of three groups:

- Inhibition of sodium conductance: these include phenytoin, carbamazepine, sodium valproate and lamotrigine

- Enhancement of GABAergic action in the CNS: this may be secondary to binding to the GABA receptor (phenobarbitone, benzodiazepines), inhibition of GABA transaminase (vigabatrin) or inhibition of GABA re-uptake (tiagabine)

- Miscellaneous: includes inhibition of calcium conductance (ethosuximide) and drugs such as gabapentin where the mode of action has not yet been determined.

1.12   C: It interacts with bendroflumethiazide (bendrofluazide)

Lithium is used for the treatment of bipolar depression and for the prophylaxis of unipolar depression. It does not affect mood in normal individuals. It is handled like sodium by the body and is excreted via the kidneys. Therefore, its use should be avoided in patients with moderate to severe renal impairment. It is also excreted in breast milk and its use should be avoided in breastfeeding mothers. It has a narrow therapeutic index, and its levels need to be monitored. Its renal excretion can be affected by non-steroidal anti-infammatory drugs (NSAIDs) and diuretics, which can precipitate lithium toxicity. Adverse effects include goitre, hypothyroidism, tremor, convulsions and nephrogenic diabetes insipidus.

1.13   C: Atenolol

An acute attack of gout should be treated with high-dose NSAIDs or colchicine. Commencement of therapy for chronic gout with drugs such as allopurinol or uricosurics such as ˙probenecid, if not covered by NSAIDs, can sometimes precipitate an acute attack. Aspirin and salicylates antagonise the uricosuric drugs and should therefore be avoided in patients with gout. Other drugs which can cause hyperuricaemia include diuretics, adenosine, ciclosporin, inosine pranobex, and alcohol.

1.14   E: Clarithromycin is active against atypical mycobacteria

Clindamycin penetrates bone well and is active against *Staphylococcus aureus,* which means it can be used in the treatment of osteomyelitis. It is particularly liable to cause pseudomembranous colitis. Methicillin-resistant *S. aureus* (MRSA or 'superbugs') have attracted media attention recently. In most cases, MRSA can be eliminated by topical therapy. Systemic therapy is only required when systemic infection is suspected: teicoplanin may be effective in such cases. Co-amoxiclav and flucloxacillin can cause cholestatic hepatitis which can appear up to six weeks after stopping the drug. The liver toxicity is thought to be due to clavulanic acid rather than amoxycillin. Clarithromycin, a macrolide, is often used in HIV-positive patients as prophylaxis against atypical mycobacteria.

1.15   C: Bioequivalence studies are usually single-dose studies

Manufacturers of generic drugs are required by law to show that their drug is bioequivalent to the brand leader. That is, the generic drug must be absorbed at the same rate and to the same extent as the brand leader. A drug can be categorised as being bioequivalent if it is shown that the absorption is within ± 20% of the branded product. The specified range is narrower for drugs such as warfarin which have a narrow therapeutic index. Bioequivalent studies are usually performed in volunteers and are single-dose studies. Bioequivalence is difficult to demonstrate with modified-release preparations, which should be prescribed by brand name. Different brands of drugs such as lithium, ciclosporin, phenytoin and other narrow therapeutic index drugs vary widely in bioavailability and should also be prescribed by brand name. However, many of the widely used drugs, such as aspirin, atenolol, bendroflumethiazide (bendrofluazide), prednisolone and amoxicillin, to name a few, can be prescribed generically.

1.16   B: Zero-order kinetics means that the rate of elimination of the drug is dependent on the plasma concentration

A first-pass effect means that the drug is extensively metabolised before it reaches the systemic circulation. As a result, drugs with a high first-pass effect have low bioavailability. Most drugs exhibit first-order kinetics but some drugs exhibit zero-order kinetics, which means that there may be a disproportionate increase in serum concentration for a small increment in dose. The terminal half-life of a drug refers to the time required to excrete half of a given dose. Glucuronidation increases the water-solubility of a drug.

1.17   D: It is treated with phenytoin

Digoxin is a drug with a narrow therapeutic index. Toxicity (even when levels are within the therapeutic range) can be precipitated by hypokalaemia, hypomagnesaemia and hypercalcaemia. Changes in the plasma sodium concentration have no effect on digoxin toxicity *per se*. Digoxin toxicity may manifest with symptoms such as nausea, vomiting, xanthopsia, or ECG changes such as ST depression (reversed tick pattern) or cardiac arrhythmias. Phenytoin can be used to treat digoxin-induced cardiac arrhythmias.

1.18   B: It can only be used in amyotrophic lateral sclerosis

The cause of motor neurone disease (MND) is unknown. It has been postulated that excitotoxic neurotransmitters such as glutamate may be involved in the pathogenesis of MND. Riluzole antagonises the effects of glutamate on nerve cells by inhibiting its release and protecting cells from glutamate-mediated damage. It has been licensed 'to extend life or the time to mechanical ventilation for patients with amyotrophic lateral sclerosis'. It is not licensed for use in other forms of MND, such as progressive muscular atrophy and progressive bulbar palsy. Riluzole has a modest effect on mortality in patients with amyotrophic lateral sclerosis but there is no evidence that it improves either functional capacity or quality of life. Riluzole causes an elevation of liver enzymes in approximately 1% of patients.

1.19   D: Atenolol

Drugs can cause anaemia by various mechanisms:

- Increased blood loss from the gastrointestinal tract: aspirin, NSAIDs, meloxicam and alendronate
- Increased red cell breakdown secondary to haemolysis: this may be metabolic (eg G6PD deficiency: sulphonamides, primaquine, nitrofurantoin) or autoimmune (nomifensine, methyldopa)
- Deficiency of vitamin B_{12} or folic acid leading to megaloblastic anaemia: metformin and methotrexate
- Bone marrow toxicity (aplastic anaemia) from drugs such as chloramphenicol, phenylbutazone, carbamazepine and felbamate.

1.20   E: Insulin receptors are linked to transmembrane protein tyrosine kinases

Drugs produce their actions by acting upon receptors, ion channels and enzymes. Most receptors are present on the plasma membrane, although oestrogen and steroid receptors are located within the cytosol and nucleus. Receptors interacting with G proteins can either modulate adenylate cyclase activity or activate phospholipase C. Insulin acts on cells by interacting with a receptor which has an extracellular hormone-binding domain and a cytoplasmic enzyme domain with protein tyrosine kinase activity. When tissues are continuously exposed to an agonist the numbers of receptors decrease or there is receptor desensitisation: this may cause tachyphylaxis (loss of efficacy with repeated doses).

1.21   C: Long-term therapy with omeprazole without antibiotics can alter the distribution of infection within the stomach

Patients with peptic ulcer who are infected with *Helicobacter pylori* have been shown to benefit from eradication therapy. However, there is little evidence that patients with non-specific dyspepsia will benefit from treatment with antibiotics. The use of antisecretory drugs in *H. pylori*-infected patients reverses the predominantly antral pattern of gastritis and increases the severity of corpus gastritis. The pattern of gastritis then resembles that more commonly associated with the development of mucosal atrophy. There is accumulating epidemiological evidence suggesting an association between *H. pylori* infection and cancer of the gastric corpus and antrum (but not of the duodenum). Eradication therapy, of which there are numerous regimens, generally has a success rate in excess of 90%.

1.22   C: It can lead to bone marrow suppression

Patients who are HCV-RNA-positive with chronic hepatitis on biopsy should be considered for treatment with interferon-α. Normalisation of serum transaminases is seen in 50% of patients but in half of these, transaminase levels rise again after stopping therapy. The sustained response rate is 15–25%; those individuals most likely to develop severe liver disease may be the least likely to respond to antiviral treatment. Treatment is contraindicated in patients with autoimmune disease, active psychiatric disorder, alcohol abuse, decompensated liver disease and pregnancy. Fever, headache and myalgia (which can be alleviated by pre-treatment with paracetamol), anorexia and fatigue are common side-effects, while bone marrow suppression, alopecia, seizures, retinopathy and psychosis are rarer adverse effects.

1.23   D: They are contra-indicated in patients with bilateral renal artery stenosis

Angiotensin-II receptor antagonists such as losartan (like ACE inhibitors) can be used in the treatment of hypertension and heart failure. Evidence suggests that they are as effective as ACE inhibitors in these conditions. Angiotensin-II receptor antagonists, however, do not block the degradation of bradykinin and are therefore less likely to cause cough and angio-oedema. Like ACE inhibitors, they are contraindicated in pregnancy and in patients with bilateral renal artery stenosis.

1.24   E: Treatment with ceftriaxone is superior to treatment with cefuroxime

Benzylpenicillin should be administered immediately in patients with suspected meningococcal disease. Studies investigating the utility of steroids have largely been performed in patients with meningitis caused by either *H. influenzae* or *Pneumococcus*: steroids have generally reduced the frequency of adverse neurological outcomes, including deafness. However, the use of steroids has not been adequately studied in patients with meningococcal meningitis and the routine use, particularly in septicaemia, cannot be recommended at present. Chemoprophylaxis with rifampicin or ciprofloxacin is indicated for household and/or intimate contacts, but not for health-care workers unless they have given mouth-to-mouth resuscitation or inhaled respiratory secretions. Third-generation cephalosporins are the mainstay of treatment in all forms of bacterial meningitis in all age groups. Cefuroxime, however, has been shown to be inferior to ceftriaxone and should not be used.

1.25   A: Tinnitus

Tinnitus and deafness are seen in salicylate poisoning of any severity. Salicylates directly stimulate the respiratory centre to increase the depth and rate of respiration, causing a respiratory alkalosis. A variable degree of metabolic acidosis is also present because of the loss of bicarbonate. Increased tissue glycolysis and increased peripheral demand for glucose can cause hypoglycaemia. Salicylates have a warfarin-like action on the vitamin K_1-epoxide cycle and can lead to hypoprothrombinaemia. Peptic ulceration is a feature of chronic salicylate therapy and not of acute poisoning.

1.26   E: It has an insidious onset

Neuroleptic malignant syndrome is an idiosyncratic reaction to therapeutic doses of phenothiazines, thioxanthines or butyrophenones. It develops insidiously over one to three days, and is characterised by hyperthermia, muscle rigidity, impaired consciousness and tachycardia and elevated creatine phosphokinase (CPK) levels. Dantrolene, but not calcium-channel blockers, may be of value. The mechanism responsible for the condition is unknown.

1.27   D: Propafenone has α-adrenoceptor-blocking activity

Adenosine is of little use in atrial fibrillation. Digoxin toxicity can lead to most types of arrhythmias, including atrial fibrillation. Digoxin is of use in chronic atrial fibrillation but not in paroxysmal atrial fibrillation. Sotalol has both class II and class III antiarrhythmic properties, and can be used in both ventricular and supraventricular tachycardias. Propafenone is a class Ic drug with actions on sodium channels, calcium channels and β-blocking activity. QT-interval prolongation may lead to *torsades de pointes*, which is difficult to treat with other antiarrhythmics, but may respond to magnesium. Magnesium has no effect on atrial fibrillation.

1.28   A: Rifabutin and clarithromycin

Zidovudine and aciclovir are often used together in patients with AIDS without causing any harmful effects. Aspirin and streptokinase were shown in the ISIS-2 study to have a beneficial effect in patients with acute myocardial infarction. Naproxen and penicillamine are often used together in patients with rheumatoid arthritis. Rifabutin metabolism can be inhibited by clarithromycin, which may result in anterior uveitis. Atenolol is commonly used together with isosorbide mononitrate in patients with angina.

1.29   B: All serious ADRs should be reported

The spontaneous adverse drug reaction (ADR) reporting scheme in the UK is called the yellow card scheme. Reporting is voluntary; it is recommended that all serious ADRs and all ADRs to new drugs (marked by ▼ in the *BNF*) should be reported. Doctors, dentists, coroners and, more recently, pharmacists are allowed to report on yellow cards. It has been estimated that only 10% of all serious ADRs and 3–4% of all ADRs are actually reported: such gross under-reporting means that the yellow card data cannot be used to estimate the frequency of a particular ADR. Yellow card reports provide a signal that a drug may have the propensity to cause a particular ADR: this can provide the impetus to initiate further epidemiological studies to allow a causal relationship to be established between an ADR and a drug.

1.30   E: Vd can be calculated from a knowledge of the dose and concentration in plasma if the drug demonstrates linear kinetics

Distribution volume is the volume of fluid in which the drug appears to distribute with a concentration equal to that in plasma. It can be calculated from a knowledge of the dose and concentration as long as the drug demonstrates linear kinetics. For example, for a drug which remains within the circulation, the distribution volume will be similar to the blood volume, ie five litres. The distribution volume can be significantly higher than that of body water if the drugs are distributed mainly within peripheral tissues. For example, the volume of distribution of chloroquine is 13,000 litres. Drugs with a low Vd, such as aspirin, are mainly within the plasma and thus can be removed by haemodialysis, particularly in overdose situations.

1.31   A: Vitamin B$_6$ status can be assessed by the tryptophan loading test

The tryptophan loading test can be used to assess vitamin B$_6$ status, except in patients receiving oestrogens or with increased secretion of corticosteroids. Vitamin B$_6$ deficiency can be induced by penicillamine and isoniazid (which increases urinary excretion). Cycloserine and hydralazine are antagonists of vitamin B$_6$. The liver plays a major role in the metabolism of pyridoxine. Pyridoxine can be used in pregnant women, for example in patients with hyperemesis gravidarum. Pyridoxine should not be given to patients receiving L-dopa as the action of L-dopa is antagonised. However, the vitamin can be used if the preparation contains both L-dopa and the dopa decarboxylase inhibitor carbidopa. High doses of pyridoxine may lead to sensory nerve damage and be manifested as paraesthesiae: this is reversible on stopping vitamin B$_6$.

1.32   D: Iodide can cause a goitre in euthyroid patients

The mainstay of treatment of thyrotoxicosis are the thionamides (carbimazole and propylthiouracil). Both inhibit the iodination of tyrosine and coupling of iodotyrosines. In addition, propylthiouracil, but not carbimazole, inhibits the peripheral conversion of T_4 to T_3. It usually takes four to eight weeks for these drugs to have an effect. In that time, β-blockers are useful: they block the adrenergic effects of excess thyroid hormone, such as sweating and tremor, but have no effect on basal metabolic rate. In euthyroid subjects an excess of iodide from any source can cause a goitre. Radioactive iodine emits mainly β radiation (90%) which penetrates only 0.5 mm of tissue. It does emit some of the more penetrating γ rays which can be detected with a Geiger counter.

1.33   E: Ethanol prevents methanol toxicity by inhibiting its oxidation within the liver

Methanol is eliminated in humans by oxidation to formaldehyde, formic acid and carbon dioxide. This is catalysed by the enzyme alcohol dehydrogenase. Blurred vision with a clear sensorium occurs 8–36 hours after poisoning, although optic atrophy is a late finding. Blood methanol levels should be determined as soon as possible. Methanol levels in excess of 50 mg/dl are thought to be an absolute indication for haemodialysis and ethanol treatment. The latter inhibits methanol oxidation by competing for alcohol dehydrogenase. Patients with methanol poisoning usually have a metabolic acidosis with an elevated anion gap.

1.34   D: Metronidazole

Drugs that inhibit the oxidation of acetaldehyde can cause a systemic reaction if taken with alcohol. This is the basis for the use of disulfiram as aversive treatment for alcoholism. Metronidazole can also inhibit acetaldehyde oxidation and tinidazole may have the same effect. Other drugs which can lead to flushing with alcohol include procarbazine, chlorpropamide, ketoconazole and cefamandole. Naltrexone is used in the treatment of alcoholics.

1.35   A: *Escherichia coli*

Resistance to antibiotics is increasing largely because of the indiscriminate, widespread and inappropriate use of antibiotics. In general, resistance to penicillins is seen in more than 20% of isolates of MRSA, *E. coli*, *Enterobacter* and *Acinetobacter* species. Resistance is unknown in β-haemolytic streptococci and *N. meningitidis*. Less than 20% of isolates of *Pseudomonas*, *N. gonorrhoeae*, *H. influenzae* and *S. pneumoniae* are resistant to penicillins.

1.36   A: Weaker inhibitors of thrombin

Low molecular weight heparins (LMWHs) have mean molecular weights in the range of 4–6 kDa. Compared to unfractionated heparin (UFH), they are weaker inhibitors of thrombin (factor IIa), but inhibit the coagulation enzyme Xa to a similar extent. Elimination of LMWHs is mainly via the kidneys and is therefore likely to be reduced in patients with renal failure. Current evidence suggests that the risk of bleeding is similar with both sets of compounds. Immune-mediated thrombocytopenia occurs with both LMWH and UFH; the risk may be lower with LMWH although this needs to be confirmed in larger studies. The osteopenic effect of LMWH may be less than that of UFH.

1.37   B: Corticosteroid replacement is necessary in patients on aminoglutethimide

In post-menopausal women, peripheral tissues are the main site of oestrogen production, usually by conversion of androstenedione and testosterone by aromatase to oestrone and oestradiol. These extraglandular sites of oestrogen production can be inhibited by aromatase inhibitors. Aminoglutethimide was the first of these inhibitors but was rather non-specific, causing inhibition of adrenal cortical enzymes as well. This necessitated the use of corticosteroid replacement. Anastrazole is a new-generation aromatase inhibitor that is more potent and highly selective. As a result it does not affect adrenal function.

1.38   B: Heart valve regurgitation has been shown to be associated with treatment with fenfluramine and phentermine

Various drugs have been used for the treatment of obesity with varying degrees of success. Appetite suppressants such as fenfluramine and phentermine have been associated with primary pulmonary hypertension and, more recently, with valvular heart disease. Although the prevalence of aortic and mitral regurgitation has varied in different studies, there is a consensus that these appetite suppressants lead to valvular heart disease (regurgitation rather than stenosis). The mechanism is unknown but may be related to increased production of serotonin (akin to the valve lesions seen in carcinoid syndrome). There is no evidence at the time of publication of this book that SSRIs (which are used for treatment of obesity) also lead to valvular heart disease. Sibutramine is a relatively new anti-obesity agent that increases blood pressure – frequent monitoring is required in patients: because of this it is also contraindicated in patients with hypertension.

1.39   A: Trazodone

Priapism is a prolonged and painful erection that cannot be relieved by sexual fulfilment. It has been reported in association with:

- phenothiazines, including chlorpromazine, promazine and fluphenazine
- the butyrophenone haloperidol
- trazodone but not conventional tricyclic antidepressants
- α-adrenoceptor antagonists, including prazosin, phenoxybenzamine and labetalol
- warfarin
- intracavernosal papaverine.

1.40   C: Desferrioxamine

The following antidotes can be used in patients with acute poisoning:

Oral anticoagulants	Vitamin K
Benzodiazepines	Flumazenil
β-blockers	Atropine
	Glucagon
Carbon monoxide	Oxygen
Cyanide	Oxygen
	Dicobalt edetate
	Hydroxocobalamin
	Sodium thiosulphate
	Sodium nitrite
Digoxin	Digoxin-specific antibody fragments
Ethylene glycol	Ethanol
	Fomepizole
Ferrous sulphate/ fumarate and other salts	Desferrioxamine
Methanol	Ethanol
Opioids	Naloxone
Organophosphates	Atropine
	Pralidoxime
Paracetamol	N-acetylcysteine

1.41   B: Decrease in gut motility

Stimulation of the α-adrenoceptor leads to vasoconstriction of most vessels in the body, in particular in the skin, mucosae, abdominal viscera and coronary circulation. Further actions include decrease in gut motility, contraction of the pregnant uterus, decreased exocrine secretion by pancreatic acini and contraction of the radial muscle of the iris. Cholinergic activity and nitric oxide are largely responsible for penile erection.

1.42   C: Increased release of virus from cells

Zanamivir is a neuraminidase inhibitor, and is licensed for the treatment of influenza A or B within 48 hours of the onset of symptoms. Neuraminidase in the virus breaks down N-acetylneuraminic acid in respiratory secretions; this allows the virus to penetrate to the surfaces of cells. Inhibition of the neuraminidase prevents infection and, in some cases, complications such as otitis media. Neuraminidase is also necessary for the optimal release of virus from infected cells, an action that increases the spread of virus and the intensity of the infection. Inhibition of neuraminidase decreases the likelihood of illness and reduces the severity of any illness that does develop. Zanamivir is inhaled through the mouth; the majority of the drug ends up in the oropharynx; overall, the drug is only 10–20% bioavailable. Zanamivir can decrease bronchial airflow, and should be used with caution in patients with chronic respiratory disease in whom it can induce clinically significant bronchospasm.

1.43   B: Can cause neutropenia and thrombocytopenia

Cephalosporins, like the penicillins, have a β-lactam ring. There is therefore a 20% risk of cross-sensitivity between the two groups: if a patient has had a severe reaction to penicillin such as anaphylaxis, then cephalosporins should either not be used at all or with extreme caution. Most cephalosporins have half-lives less than three hours. Cephalosporins are associated with a number of adverse effects, including skin rashes, anaphylaxis, neutropenia and thrombocytopenia, and are one of the most important causes of *Clostridium difficile* diarrhoea. Indeed, the current epidemic of *Clostridium difficile* diarrhoea has been blamed on the British Thoracic Society guidelines that recommended the use of cephalosporins in the treatment of community-acquired pneumonia.

1.44   D: Sarcoidosis

The hypercalcaemia of sarcoidosis responds to steroids better than the other causes listed. Irrespective of the cause of hypercalcaemia, the first choice of treatment should always be rehydration with normal saline. Furosemide (frusemide) used concomitantly does not provide a better calcium-reducing effect. Only when patients have been rehydrated should bisphosphonates be used.

1.45   A: Approximately 8% of the population cannot convert codeine to morphine

Morphine is the drug of choice for controlling severe forms of pain. It is available in various formulations, including:

- Normal-release: onset of action 20 minutes; peak drug levels 60 minutes
- Twice-daily controlled-release preparations: onset of action 1–2 hours; peak drug levels at 4 hours
- Once-daily controlled-release preparation: slower onset of action with peak drug levels at 8.5 hours.

Both diamorphine and codeine are pro-drugs, being converted to morphine in the body. Diamorphine is more soluble than morphine. Codeine is converted to morphine by the P450 enzyme CYP2D6, which is polymorphically expressed, being absent in 8–10% of the population. Many of the effects of morphine are subject to the phenomenon of tolerance, including the analgesic and euphoric effects. Importantly, miosis is not subject to tolerance and can be used as a sign to indicate opiate misuse.

1.46   C: Drugs with intrinsic sympathomimetic activity are less likely to cause bradycardia

Beta-blockers have many different properties, which can be used to differentiate their actions and side-effect profile. These include lipophilicity, cardioselectivity and intrinsic sympathomimetic activity (ISA). Beta-blockers with ISA are less likely to cause bradycardia. Beta-blockers such as atenolol are cardioselective but not cardiospecific: this means that they can still affect β_2 receptors, especially when used in high dosage. Beta-blockers have class II antiarrhythmic properties and, apart from sotalol (which also has class III properties), are unlikely to affect the QT interval. Celiprolol is a 'vasodilating' β-blocker and usually decreases total peripheral resistance. Esmolol is a short-acting β-blocker that is given intravenously to treat supraventricular arrhythmias.

1.47   A: Can cause selective IgA deficiency

Phenytoin is an anticonvulsant used for the treatment of generalised tonic-clonic convulsions and partial seizures. It can exacerbate myoclonic epilepsy, and can precipitate seizures when levels are high. It displays zero-order kinetics, ie due to saturation of metabolism; small changes in dose can lead to disproportionate increase in serum levels, with dose-dependent toxicity. It can cause a wide variety of adverse effects, including immune-mediated adverse reactions such as skin rashes, hepatitis and aplastic anaemia. It can also lead to other immunological abnormalities affecting both the cellular and humoral arms of the immune system. With respect to the latter, selective IgA deficiency is a well-recognised adverse reaction. Phenytoin is an enzyme inducer and can cause vitamin D deficiency, leading to osteomalacia. Phenytoin is also an antiarrhythmic, used to treat digoxin-induced arrhythmias. It can, however, also lead to rhythm abnormalities such as bradycardia and ectopic beats in 2% of patients.

1.48   A: Cimetidine and dapsone

Rifampicin is an enzyme inducer, which can lower ciclosporin levels, leading to graft rejection. This is a serious interaction that can be overcome by monitoring ciclosporin levels and increasing the dose.

Cimetidine is an enzyme inhibitor that can inhibit phenytoin metabolism, leading to phenytoin toxicity.

Ritonavir is a potent enzyme inhibitor: it can inhibit the metabolism of fluoxetine, which can lead to a potentially fatal reaction called the serotonin syndrome.

Erythromycin is an enzyme inhibitor that can affect the metabolism of cisapride: this can lead to prolongation of the QT interval and occasionally to *torsades de pointes* and sudden death.

Cimetidine is an enzyme inhibitor which is known to inhibit dapsone metabolism. However, it results in reduced formation of a toxic metabolite of dapsone: this toxic metabolite is known to cause methaemoglobinaemia. This combination has therefore been used in patients with dermatitis herpetiformis to improve the tolerability of dapsone.

1.49   A: Blood glucose > 8.3 mmol/l

Iron overdose is more common in children than in adults. Severe poisoning is characterised by haematemesis, hypotension, coma and shock. Disintegrating tablets may make the stools grey or black in colour, and this does not necessarily indicate a gastrointestinal bleed. A white cell count of > 15×10^9/l and blood glucose level > 8.3 mmol/l in the six hours after ingestion, together with the presence of tablets on abdominal X-ray, have been shown to correlate with serum iron concentrations > 54 mmol/l. A challenge dose of desferrioxamine which results in urine with a red/orange colour indicates the presence of free circulating iron, and is an indication for further treatment with desferrioxamine.

1.50   D: Rivastigmine binds to both the anionic and esteratic sites of the enzyme

Alzheimer's disease is characterised by decreased acetylcholine activity, and currently available drugs aim to increase cholinergic activity. Acetylcholine is broken down by acetylcholinesterase (AChE), and inhibition will increase acetylcholine activity. Acetylcholinesterase has both anionic and esteratic sites; its activity can be inhibited by binding to either site. Donepezil and the recently withdrawn drug tacrine, both act at the anionic site in a reversible fashion: they thus have a relatively short duration of enzyme inhibition. However, donepezil has a long half-life (70 hours) and thus only needs to be dosed once daily. Metrifonate, a pro-drug, which is converted to an active metabolite that binds irreversibly to the esteratic site of AChE was recently withdrawn because of its potential to cause respiratory paralysis. Like acetylcholine, rivastigmine binds to both the anionic and esteratic sites; it needs to be administered twice daily.

1.51   E: Vigabatrin – anterior uveitis

Cerivastatin is an HMG-CoA reductase inhibitor that is highly potent, but causes rhabdomyolysis to a greater extent than the other HMG-CoA reductase inhibitors. For this reason, it was withdrawn from the market. Indinavir is a protease inhibitor that can crystallise out in urine, particularly when concentrations in plasma are high, and may in some cases lead to renal stones. Tolcapone is a COMT inhibitor used in Parkinson's disease; it was withdrawn because of its potential to cause hepatotoxicity and neuroleptic malignant syndrome but it is to be re-introduced soon for resistant patients who have not responded to entacapone. Vigabatrin causes peripheral visual field constriction in 30% of patients: this is thought to be irreversible, and although the mechanism of the adverse effect is not known, the retina is thought to be the site of toxicity. Pergolide is a dopamine agonist, and like all drugs of this class, it can cause fibrotic reactions, including pulmonary fibrosis, pleural fibrosis and retroperitoneal fibrosis.

1.52   E: It inhibits purine synthesis

Leflunomide is a disease-modifying antirheumatic drug, like gold, penicillamine, chloroquine, ciclosporin, sulfasalazine, methotrexate and azathioprine. Leflunomide inhibits pyrimidine synthesis through inhibition of dihydro-orotate dehydrogenase, and is rapidly converted to an active metabolite. Its efficacy is comparable to that of sulfasalazine and methotrexate.

1.53   B: Dose requirements are genetically determined

Warfarin is an oral anticoagulant, which acts as a vitamin K antagonist by inhibiting vitamin K epoxide reductase. Dose requirements vary widely: these are at least partly determined by genetic polymorphisms affecting the P450 enzymes (CYP2C9) responsible for the metabolism of warfarin. The dose can be adjusted by monitoring the international normalised ratio (INR). Overdosage predisposes to bleeding, which can be treated with fresh frozen plasma and vitamin K. Warfarin does not affect bone density; however, osteoporosis can be caused by heparin.

1.54   A: Accidental injection of lidocaine (lignocaine) into the systemic circulation may increase myocardial and neuronal excitability

Lidocaine, an amide local anaesthetic, is commonly used for minor surgery and in dental practice. Its duration of action can be prolonged by the addition of adrenaline (epinephrine), which causes vasoconstriction. Lidocaine is shorter-acting than bupivacaine, and undergoes extensive metabolism. Intravenous injection can lead to cardiac arrhythmias and seizures.

1.55   D: The incidence of benign breast disease may be increased

Oral contraceptives contain progestogens, which inhibit LH release, while the oestrogen component inhibits FSH release. Oestrogens, particularly at high dosage, promote blood clotting: this risk is increased in women over 35 years, who are obese and smokers. Third-generation oral contraceptives have a twofold higher risk of venous thromboembolism than second-generation compounds. Thrombogenicity is also increased in patients who are carriers of the factor V Leiden mutation. There is also a small increase in the absolute risk of stroke with the oral contraceptive. The oral contraceptive pill also has many beneficial effects, including a reduced risk of benign breast disease and of ovarian cancer.

1.56   A: Does not have a beneficial effect if administered at the time of the first-ever demyelinating event

Interferon-β has demonstrated benefits in the treatment of patients with established multiple sclerosis, including slowing the progression of physical disability, reducing the rate of clinical relapses, and reducing the development of brain lesions, as assessed by MRI, and brain atrophy. A recent study has shown that initiating treatment at the time of the first demyelinating event is beneficial in patients with lesions on MRI that indicate a high risk of clinically definite multiple sclerosis.

1.57   E: Trazodone

Drug	Anticholinergic	Cardiac	Nausea effects	Sedation effects
Amitriptyline	+++	+++	+	+++
Clomipramine	+++	++	+	++
Dothiepin	++	++	-	+++
Lofepramine	++	+	+	+
Trazodone	+	+	++	++

1.58   D: It inhibits the release of calcitonin gene-related peptide

Sumatriptan does not affect the aura of migraine and should be taken as soon as the headache starts. Triptans exhibit highly selective and potent agonist activity at the 1B, 1D, 1F and 1A 5-HT receptors. Stimulation of the 5-HT_{1D} receptor inhibits CGRP release and thus dural vasodilatation. Sumatriptan should not be used in patients with ischaemic heart disease, Prinzmetal's angina or severe systemic hypertension. It should not be used with ergotamine, which can also cause coronary vasoconstriction. The drug is almost 100% bioavailable after sub-cutaneous administration, while bioavailability after oral administration is 14%.

1.59   B: It is a selective inhibitor of the neuronal uptake of noradrenaline

Bupropion (Zyban®) was initially used as an antidepressant, but has recently been licensed for smoking cessation. It inhibits the uptake of both noradrenaline and serotonin; it reduces nicotine craving and withdrawal symptoms. Patients treated with bupropion are twice as likely to have stopped smoking at one year compared with those on nicotine replacement therapy. Bupropion is associated with a large number of adverse effects: seizures occur in 1/1000 patients, while skin rashes are common, with a small number developing Stevens–Johnson syndrome. Bupropion is metabolised by a P450 enzyme called CYP2B6, but inhibits another P450 enzyme called CYP2D6, and can therefore be involved in interactions.

1.60   D: Oxcarbazepine

Hyoscine, neostigmine, codeine and propranolol are present in milk in concentrations that are too low to have a significant effect on the infant. Of the β-blockers, most are excreted in too small amounts to have an effect, but the infant should be monitored for bradycardia. Acebutolol, atenolol, nadolol and sotalol are present in greater amounts than other β-blockers. Appendix 5 of the *BNF* is a good source of information on drugs excreted in breast milk.

1.61   E: Vincristine

Vincristine is a vinca alkaloid treatment; it has no role in the treatment of minimal-change glomerulonephritis. Nephrotic syndrome due to minimal-change nephropathy is responsive to all the other agents.

1.62   A: Analgesic nephropathy was previously the commonest cause of renal failure in Australia

Analgesic nephropathy virtually always occurs after a cumulative dose of analgesics of at least 1 kg. It does not usually occur until heavy use has taken place for two years. Between 1950 and 1970, analgesic nephropathy was the commonest cause of renal failure in Australia, but has waned since phenacetin was banned. The primary renal lesion is papillary necrosis, which can also be caused by diabetes, urinary obstruction and sickle cell disease. Many patients have had successful renal transplants.

1.63   C: Analgesic nephropathy is characterised pathologically by glomerulonephritis

The renal lesion of analgesic nephropathy is papillary necrosis. Amphotericin B reduces renal blood flow and causes renal tubular acidosis.

1.64   A: Concomitant administration of diuretics makes aminoglycoside toxicity more likely

Toxicity may be avoided by dose reduction or reduced dosage frequency. Aminoglycosides require peak and trough levels for accurate estimation of potential nephrotoxicity. Aminoglycoside toxicity is more likely in a dehydrated patient or in the presence of hypokalaemia. Vancomycin is cleared renally and with renal impairment therapeutic levels can be found up to five days after a single dose; drug levels should guide further doses. All drugs reach steady state after five half-lives.

1.65   C: Nifedipine

Cholestyramine is an ion exchange resin used in the management of hypercholesterolaemia. As it is not absorbed, gastrointestinal side-effects are common, particularly constipation. The commonest side-effect of verapamil therapy is constipation. Nifedipine affects different calcium channels from those affected by verapamil and, in particular, does not affect the channels in the large bowel to the same extent. TCA and disopyramide have anticholinergic side-effects, including constipation. Thiazides may cause constipation indirectly, due to hypercalcaemia or hypokalaemia, or by dehydration.

1.66   B: Glypressin

Intravenous ranitidine is of no value in gastrointestinal haemorrhage due to varices. Antibiotics reduce mortality in those patients presenting for the first time. Octreotide reduces the risk of rebleeding, but not mortality. Propranolol is most effective for prevention of rebleeding.

1.67   A: Digoxin

Metformin is normally inactivated in the liver and should be avoided because it causes lactic acidosis. Erythromycin is associated with a risk of hepatotoxicity and should be avoided in liver failure. Digoxin is excreted unchanged by the kidneys. Propranolol undergoes extensive first-pass metabolism and this will not occur in liver disease, thus increasing the systemic availability. All opiates should be avoided because of the increased risk of coma.

1.68   A: Acute alcohol intake

Paracetamol is metabolised to a quinone-amine metabolite which is normally conjugated with glutathione. In paracetamol overdose, glutathione is depleted and the metabolite induces liver necrosis. Patients with reduced stores of glutathione are at increased risk of paracetamol toxicity, (eg malnourished patients, patients with anorexia and HIV-positive patients). Increased production of the toxic metabolite will also increase the risk of toxicity, for example patients on enzyme inducers such as phenytoin, carbamazepine and rifampicin. Isoniazid is known to be an enzyme inhibitor and inducer and has been shown to increase the risk of paracetamol toxicity. Acute alcohol intake is an enzyme inhibitor as opposed to chronic alcohol intake, which is an enzyme inducer. Despite this, it would be unwise to treat patients with a history of acute alcohol intake as low-risk as many of these patients have a history of chronic alcohol abuse.

1.69 E: Reducing nucleotide biosynthesis

Methotrexate binds to the intracellular enzyme dihydrofolate reductase. This enzyme is responsible for the production of reduced dihydrofolate, which is a co-factor involved in the synthesis of nucleotides and the amino acids serine and methionine. Methotrexate therefore interferes with nucleotide and protein synthesis. Methotrexate can be given orally or intravenously. Folinic acid is often given 24 hours after high-dose intravenous methotrexate treatment. This helps to reduce the severity of methotrexate-induced myelosuppression and mucositis.

1.70 B: Busulfan

Other cytotoxic drugs that can cause lung fibrosis include bleomycin and methotrexate. These drugs cause acute interstitial pulmonary inflammation, which results in fibrotic changes. The diagnosis of drug-induced lung fibrosis is suggested by bilateral chest X-ray (CXR) shadowing in conjunction with a restrictive defect on pulmonary function testing. The differential diagnosis in cancer patients receiving chemotherapy is of metastatic carcinoma or pulmonary infection (often atypical). The diagnosis of lung fibrosis is confirmed by high-resolution computed tomography (CT) scanning (which typically shows fibrosis and a ground-glass appearance, the latter indicating active inflammation) and bronchoscopy with transbronchial biopsy for histological examination (or biopsy by video-assisted thoracoscopy).

1.71 C: The G1 and S phases

The stages of the cell cycle begin with the G0 (latent) phase. G1 is the resting phase when the cellular components required for DNA are synthesised. Cells then enter the S phase when DNA is synthesised. Then there is the G2 (pre-mitotic) phase, leading to the M (mitosis) phase. 5-Fluorouracil inhibits the synthesis of nucleotides during late G1, so preventing the synthesis of DNA during the S phase.

1.72 D: Chronic myeloid leukaemia

Hydroxyurea is an analogue of urea. It reduces the activity of the enzyme ribonucleotide reductase, which results in the inhibition of DNA synthesis. It is mainly used in the treatment of patients with chronic myeloid leukaemia who do not receive aggressive chemotherapy regimes or bone marrow transplantation. It is administered orally. High doses may cause gastrointestinal side-effects (eg nausea, vomiting and diarrhoea). Bone marrow suppression is another possible side-effect.

1.73   B: Dapsone

Rifampicin, sulphonamides, griseofulvin, and chloroquine should not be used in people with acute intermittent porphyria (autosomal dominant inheritance). Penicillins, tetracyclines and chloramphenicol are safe to use.

1.74   D: Metformin

Insulin resistance is a state in which normal concentrations of insulin produce a subnormal biological response. Patients with insulin resistance have hyper-insulinaemia together with normoglycaemia or hyperglycaemia. It is commonly associated with obesity, non-insulin-dependent diabetes mellitus and essential hypertension. The insulin resistance syndrome includes impaired insulin-stimulated glucose uptake, hyperinsulinaemia, glucose intolerance, hypertension, and dyslipidaemia. Drugs such as corticosteroids, β-blockers, and high-dose thiazides can exacerbate insulin resistance; angiotensin-converting enzyme inhibitors and α-blockers may reduce the resistance. Other factors which can reduce insulin resistance include optimising weight, aerobic exercise, stopping smoking, and moderate alcohol consumption. Metformin improves multiple aspects of the insulin resistance syndrome. Novel insulin-enhancing drugs, including thiazolidinediones, are now increasingly important in the management of non-insulin dependent diabetes mellitus.

1.75   D: Reduces the risk of vertebral fractures by 30%

Raloxifene, a selective estrogen receptor modulator (SERM), is a non-steroidal benzothiophene, chemically related to tamoxifen. It is extensively glucuronidated in the gut wall and liver, with a mean bioavailability of the active drug of 2%. Plasma concentrations peak six hours after an oral dose and an elimination half-life of around 28 hours allows once-daily dosing. Excretion of raloxifene and its metabolites is mainly in the faeces, with less than 6% appearing in the urine. It is currently used for the prevention of non-traumatic vertebral fractures in post-menopausal women considered at increased risk of osteoporosis. It has been shown to reduce the risk of vertebral body fractures by 30%, although it has had no impact in terms of reducing the rate of non-vertebral body fractures. It does not result in post-menopausal vaginal bleeding and reduces the risk of developing breast carcinoma. It does not reduce menopausal vasomotor symptoms. Other side-effects include venous thromboembolism, thrombophlebitis, hot flushes, leg cramps and peripheral oedema.

1.76   C: Captopril

In patients with uncomplicated diabetes, hypertension may be treated initially with a low dose of a thiazide diuretic (eg 2.5 mg bendroflumethiazide daily) – in higher doses thiazides can exacerbate hyperglycaemia and dyslipidaemia. A cardioselective β-blocker such as atenolol is an alternative but can interfere with awareness of hypoglycaemia. If these fail to lower blood pressure, or if unwanted effects occur, an ACE inhibitor, calcium-channel blocker or α-blocker can be tried. In hypertensive patients with diabetic nephropathy blood pressure reduction slows the decline in renal function and ACE inhibitors are the treatment of choice, being more effective in this respect than other antihypertensive drugs.

IMMUNOLOGY: 'BEST OF FIVE' ANSWERS

2.1   C: Mixed cryoglobulinaemia

Palpable purpura with a normal platelet count suggests a vasculitis. In this context, an abnormal dipstick urinalysis suggests glomerulonephritis. Options B–E can produce this picture although it would be unusual for rheumatoid disease to present with vasculitis (without arthritis) and glomerular disease is unusual in rheumatoid.

The other notable feature is a very low C4, suggesting marked activation of the classical complement pathway. This can occur in options A, C, D, and E. but is not usually a feature of Henoch–Schönlein purpura.

Lupus is very unlikely because of the negative ANA and DNA antibodies.

The presentation is highly suggestive of mixed cryoglobulinaemia. In this syndrome, immune complexes made up of monoclonal IgM rheumatoid factor and polyclonal IgG are deposited in the tissues and cause a vasculitic process in which marked complement consumption occurs. This syndrome is strongly associated with chronic hepatitis C infection and this diagnosis is also suggested by the abnormal liver function tests. The diagnosis was confirmed by characterisation of a cryoglobulin, renal biopsy and hepatitis C serology. The patient later gave a history of intravenous drug use on a few occasions in his late teens.

2.2   B: Primary antibody deficiency

Pneumococcal infection is an unusual cause of septic arthritis. This, together with a history of chronic chest problems, suggests immunodeficiency. Antibodies are crucial for defence against capsulate bacteria such as pneumococci and *Haemophilus influenzae*, and failure to produce antibodies typically leads to infection with these organisms in the respiratory tract and elsewhere. Multiple myeloma can lead to antibody deficiency and pneumococcal infection but is very rare in this age group. Coeliac disease can be associated with a predisposition to pneumococcal infection (due to splenic atrophy) but this is usually fulminating septicaemia rather than the picture in this case. Cystic fibrosis is associated with chest and joint disease but not with pneumococcal infection. Children with HIV can have defective antibody production and are prone to pneumococcal infection in early childhood. Adults with HIV tend to present with infections suggestive of defective T cell function: infections with intracelluar organisms such as mycobacteria, fungi (eg *Candida* and *Pneumocystis*) and viruses (especially herpesviruses).

2.3   B: Neutrophil function tests

The long history of recurrent and unusual infections suggests immunodeficiency. The family history suggests a genetic cause (?X-linked). Severe/recurrent staphylococcal and fungal infection is highly suggestive of defective phagocyte function. Antibody deficiency tends to lead to recurrent infection with capsulate bacteria such as pneumococci and *Haemophilus influenzae*. T cell deficiency (whether genetic, HIV-induced or secondary to immunosuppressive drug treatment) leads particularly to infections with intracellular organisms such as mycobacteria, fungi (eg *Candida* and *Pneumocystis*), and viruses (especially herpesviruses). The history suggests a genetic cause, but no common chromosomal defects cause this picture and karyotyping is unlikely to help. Syndromes of abnormal ciliary function (such as Kartagener's syndrome) can present with chronic lung disease but these organisms and the invasive infections would be unusual. The picture is therefore highly suggestive of a genetic disorder of neutrophil function, and in particular chronic granulomatous disease, which can present in adults, although usually with a history of childhood ill-health. This syndrome is caused by a number of genetic defects (some X-linked, some autosomal recessive) which all lead to a failure of the respiratory burst in phagocytic cells. A variety of neutrophil function tests are available, the most widely known being the nitroblue tetrazolium (NBT) test.

2.4   C: Cross-linking of antigen-specific IgE bound to high-affinity IgE receptors

The patient's history suggests peanut-induced anaphylaxis. Patients with type I hypersensitivity to peanut produce IgE antibodies against peanut antigens. A T helper 2 (TH2) T cell response against peanut antigens drives this kind of antibody production. The tendency to produce this kind of immune response is in part genetic and is associated with a tendency to produce high levels of IgE against many common environmental antigens and a high level of IgE overall (this tendency is known as atopy). However, these IgE antibodies will not cause harm unless the patient is exposed to the appropriate antigen. IgE binds with high affinity to the surface of mast cells. If peanut-specific IgE bound to the surface of mast cells recognises the appropriate nut antigen, then this will cause cross-linking of the IgE receptors which leads to degranulation of the mast cells. The mediators released, such as histamine, cause the clinical features of anaphylaxis. Mast cell tryptase is released by degranulation of mast cells but does not play a major role in the anaphylactic reaction. Detection of mast cell tryptase can, however, be clinically useful in making a diagnosis of anaphylaxis in a patient who has collapsed without an obvious cause (and can be used to make a post-mortem diagnosis of anaphylaxis).

Activation of the sympathetic nervous system will occur as a response to anaphylaxis and is not the cause.

2.5   D: Addison's Disease

This woman has a clinical picture highly suggestive of an autoimmune polyendocrine syndrome (APS). Two types of APS have been described which show different patterns of incidence of endocrine dysfunction:

APS type I

Hypoparathyroidism	> 80%
Addison's disease	60–70%
Type 1 diabetes	10%
Thyroid disease	10–40%
Pernicious anaemia	10%
Gonadal failure	50% women, 10% men

There is almost always a background of chronic mucocutaneous candidiasis. Inheritance is usually autosomal recessive. APS type 1 is now also known as **a**utoimmune **p**oly**e**ndocrinopathy **c**andidiasis **e**ctodermal **d**ystrophy (APECED). Mutations in the *AIRE* gene are the cause of most cases of this syndrome.

APS type II

Type 1 diabetes	50%
Thyroid disease	70%
Addison's disease	70%
Gonadal failure	5% women, 30% men
Myasthenia gravis	1%
Pernicious anaemia	< 1%
Coeliac disease	2–5%

The patient referred to in this case has type II APS, sometimes known as Schmidt's syndrome. This can show an autosomal dominant pattern of inheritance with variable penetrance.

2.6   D: Interleukin-2 (IL-2) and interferon-γ (IFN-γ)

T cells are classed on the basis of CD4 or CD8 surface antigen expression, and on the production of cytokines. In the mouse two types of helper T cells, TH1 and TH2, are associated with cell-mediated and humoural immunity respectively. The TH1 cells secrete interleukin-2 (IL-2) and interferon-γ, and TH2 cells IL-4 and IL-10. Most human T-cells have both TH1 and TH2 activity.

Interleukins-2 and -15 induce T-cell proliferation and IL-4 and -13 (both also secreted by T cells) encourage B-cell activation and proliferation. T cells also produce the endothelial activator TNF-β.

Macropahges secrete tumour necrosis factor-α, IL-1, and IL-8. They also produce IL-10 (as do T cells), and IL-12 (as do B cells). Tumour necrosis factor-α regulates cell growth and stimulates leucocytes and adhesion receptor induction.

Transforming growth factor-β (TGF-β) is a product of T cells and monocytes. It promotes humoural immunity, reducing the acute inflammatory reaction and inhibiting cell growth.

Interferon-α and -β are produced principally by leucocytes and fibroblasts respectively, and induce adaptations in unaffected cells that increase protection against viral invasion.

2.7   B: B cell/bone marrow

Immune surveillance or 'tolerance' is an important process that reduces auto-reactivity to 'self'. Both primary (central) and secondary (peripheral) processes prevent auto-reactivity. For B cells this occurs initially in the bone marrow and then peripherally in the spleen and lymph nodes. A peripheral mechanism is required because B cells can continue to change and possibly express new immunoglobulins that are reactive to 'self'. The T-cell receptor does not undergo similar changes peripherally and therefore has only a central site of regulation, which is in the thymus.

2.8   B: DiGeorge syndrome

Primary immunodeficiency disorders tend to occur in childhood and are most often X-linked. Examples A, C and E are B-cell defects. Patients with Wiskott–Aldrich syndrome (often manifest as thrombocytopenia and lymphopenia) and severe combined immunodeficieny have B-cell and T-cell defects. Ataxia telangiectasia is another condition associated with several deficiencies of immunoglobulins and lymphopenia. The DiGeorge syndrome is a T-cell disorder, as are purine nucleoside phosphorylase deficiency and Bloom's syndrome. Other primary deficiencies of immunoregulation include complement receptor-3 deficiencies and the phagocyte disorders (eg myeloperoxidase deficiency, Job's syndrome and Chediak–Higashi syndrome).

Secondary immunodeficiency is much more common than primary disease and causes include therapies (chemotherapeutic drugs, corticosteroids, irradiation, plasmapheresis), viral infections (HIV, influenza), malignancies (solid tumours, lymphoproliferative disorders), autoimmune rheumatic diseases (systemic lupus erythematosus, dermatomyositis, vasculitis, rheumatoid arthritis), diabetes mellitus and poor nutrition.

2.9   A: Hepatitis C

Cryoglobulins are immunoglobulins that precipitate at a temperature of 40 °C. There are three categories of cryoglobulin, type I monoclonal immunoglobulin, type II mixed monoclonal/polyclonal, and type III polyclonal immunoglobulin. Type I disorders include examples B and E. Type III disorders include examples C and D. Hepatitis C, Sjögren's syndrome, and lymphoproliferative disorders are associated with type II cryoglobulinaemia.

Common clinical manifestations of cryoglobulinaemia include arthralgia, cutaneous vasculitis, hepatitis, and muscle weakness (rarely myositis). Rarer complaints include Raynaud's phenomenon, hyperviscosity syndrome, and neuropathies.

2.10   A: The Fab portion of one heavy chain linked to one light chain

A Fab fragment is monovalent and is generated by papain digestion of immunoglobulin. The Fab fragment is made up of an intact light chain and the N-terminal variable and constant H1 domains of the heavy chain.

INFECTIOUS DISEASES: 'BEST OF FIVE'
ANSWERS

3.1   B: gp41

The viral gp41 glycoprotein is involved in fusion of the virus envelope to the host cell membrane. Enfuvirtide is the first licensed fusion inhibitor and works by binding and blocking gp41. The gp120 glycoprotein on the surface of the virus binds the CD4 molecule on the T cell. CCR5 and CXCR4 are chemokine receptors on the cell surface and act as co-receptors for HIV binding. Patients with mutations in these molecules (particularly those homozygous for the Delta32 mutation of CCR5) tend to have slower progression of their HIV disease. The p24 protein is a structural protein of the core of the virion.

3.2   A: Prion protein is encoded on the host genome

Prion protein is encoded on the host genome and the amino acid sequence varies between species. Normal prion protein is produced and cleared in normal individuals. Abnormal prion protein, however, accumulates, leading to plaque formation surrounded by spongiform change. Glycosylation patterns are similar between BSE prion protein and vCJD prion protein. Patients homozygous for methionine or valine at codon 129 of the prion protein are at greater risk of more rapid disease progression. Infectivity of abnormal prion protein can be reduced and abolished by proteolytic enzymes, but not by standard sterilisation or nucleases. Tonsillar biopsy is useful in the diagnosis of variant CJD but not sporadic CJD.

3.3   D: Yellow fever vaccine

Yellow fever vaccine is a live attenuated vaccine and has caused fatal disease in patients with very advanced HIV disease. Small studies have suggested that it is probably safe in patients whose HIV is not advanced. The other vaccines are either killed or subunit vaccines. Their efficacy is very much lower in patients with advanced HIV but they are otherwise safe.

3.4   E: Hepatitis C

The list of statutory notifiable diseases can be found in the *British National Formulary*. There are many surprising omissions from this list, which appears rather out of date. Viral hepatitis is the only one of the five answers given that is on the list.

3.5   D: Rectal biopsy

This man has schistosomiasis, which is endemic in the great lakes of Africa. Some six weeks after exposure patients may develop a fever, eosinophilia and urticaria (Katayama fever). At this time patients infected with *Schistosoma mansoni* may develop a frank colitis due to a vigorous granulomatous reaction around the eggs making their way out through the wall of the colon. Diagnosis is by microscopy for ova, either in the stool for *S. mansoni* or urine for *S. haematobium*. Eggs of either species may be seen by low-power microscopy of rectal biopsies. Antibodies against *Schistosoma* species can be detected but may take up to three months from exposure to develop. The drug of choice is praziquantel.

African trypanosomiasis (*Trypanosoma brucei varrhodesiense* or *gambiense*) is transmitted by the bite of the tsetse fly and causes and acute febrile illness and subsequently sleeping sickness. There is no eosinophilia. Amoebic dysentery and amoebic liver abscesses cause a neutrophilia. Filarial infections do cause an eosinophilia, but not bloody diarrhoea.

3.6   B: Doxycycline

He has African tick typhus (*Rickettsia africae*) which is an extremely common infection, particularly amongst visitors to game parks. Sero-epidemiological studies of local people show extremely high rates of past infection. Typically, a black scab (eschar) forms at the site of the tick bite, the patient becomes febrile and complains of a severe headache and may develop a very sparse maculopapular rash. The condition is normally self-limiting but the clinical course is shortened by treatment with doxycycline. Diagnosis is usually made by testing acute and convalescent sera for a rise in specific antibody titre. Culture of the organism is hazardous for laboratory staff. Praziquantel is used in the treatment of schistosomiasis, sodium stibogluconate for leishmaniasis, and melarsoprol for African trypanosomiasis

3.7   B: *Chlamydia trachomatis*

This man has urethritis, presumably of infectious origin. Recurrent herpes simplex can occasionally affect the urethra. The negative Gram stain does not exclude gonorrhoea but it is more likely that he has non-specific urethritis (non-gonococcal urethritis), the commonest cause of which is *C. trachomatis*. It is unlikely that a primary syphilitic chancre would cause urethritis, and it is likely it would be noticed on examination. Although he claims to be monogamous, his partner may not be.

3.8   D: Yellow fever

All of these illnesses are transmitted by the bite of a mosquito. Yellow fever is present in South America and sub-Saharan Africa, but is not present in Asia or Southeast Asia although the mosquito vectors of the these areas seem capable of transmitting it in experimental situations. Dengue fever causes huge epidemics in the tropics and is frequently seen as a cause of fever in the returning traveller. *W. bancrofti* and *P. vivax* are widely distributed throughout the tropics. Japanese encephalitis has a wide distribution throughout Asia.

3.9   E: Persistent, uncontrolled infection can occur as an X-linked condition in males

This is acute Epstein–Barr virus (EBV) infection. Persistent uncontrolled EBV infection does occur very rarely and can be diagnosed by detecting high levels of EBV DNA in the blood. It is presumed that these patients have a hitherto unsuspected immunological deficit leading to the failure to control the virus. X-linked proliferative syndrome (XLP, Duncan's syndrome) is a congenital syndrome of failure to control EBV. The atypical lymphocytes are CD-8 T lymphocytes. The Paul–Bunnell test detects the presence of heterophile antibodies which do not appear to be directed against any EBV antigens. The tonsillar enlargement may be severe enough to cause respiratory embarrassment and should be treated with intravenous steroids. A fine maculopapular rash is very common. A much more dramatic rash is seen when the patient is given amoxicillin (including in co-amoxiclav) or ampicillin, which should therefore be avoided.

3.10   B: Treatment with a nucleoside reverse transcriptase inhibitor may be indicated

About 10% of people fail to respond adequately to hepatitis B vaccine. Surgeons who fail to respond to vaccination should be checked for hepatitis B acquisition every six months. Health-care workers who are HBsAg-positive, HBeAg-positive cannot be involved in exposure-prone procedures. Health-care workers who are HBsAg-positive, HBeAg-negative must have their hepatitis B DNA viral load measured and if greater than 1000 copies/ml cannot be involved in exposure and procedures. A detailed history should be taken from the surgeon to find out if there are other risk factors for hepatitis B acquisition outside the work setting. Hepatitis B immunoglobulin, if it is to be given, should be given ideally within 48 hours and certainly within a week of exposure. Lamivudine, a nucleoside reverse transcriptase inhibitor used in HIV treatment, is licensed for treatment of hepatitis B (hepatitis B undergoes a reverse transcription phase in its replication cycle).

3.11   D: The illness is highly unlikely to be acute pulmonary histoplasmosis

Although this woman is from the right area of the USA to have contracted histoplasmosis, the incubation period of acute pulmonary histoplasmosis is one to three weeks. Blood cultures are only positive in 10–30% of patients with *S. pneumoniae* pneumonia, pneumococcal urinary antigen detection being a much more sensitive test. Serology for any acute respiratory infection is likely to be negative early in illness and is best detected some two to four weeks after the onset of symptoms. *Legionella* urinary antigen testing only detects *Legionella pneumophila* type 1, which does account for 70% or more of infections. Cold agglutinins (detectable at the bedside by cooling blood in an EDTA bottle and then examining visually for red cell agglutination) are virtually diagnostic of *Mycoplasma*, the only other common condition producing cold agglutinins at this level being non-Hodgkin's lymphoma.

3.12   A: Brucellosis

Brucellosis is caused by a Gram-negative cocco-bacillus which grows reasonably quickly by modern blood culture techniques. *Coxiella burnetii* (the causative agent of Q fever) does not grow in blood culture. RVF and CCHF are both viral infections transmitted by direct blood contact and possibly also by mosquitoes (RVF) and tick bites (CCHF). In acute sleeping sickness (*Trypanosoma brucei* var *gambiense* or *rhodesiense*) the trypanosomes are often visible on a thick blood film, but sleeping sickness does not occur in the Middle East. The other four illnesses do occur, especially in people in close contact with herds of sheep and goats, with brucellosis and Q fever being more common than the other two diseases.

3.13   A: *Candida albicans*

Prolonged stay in an intensive care unit is associated with an increased risk of *Candida* septicaemia and this is by far the most likely diagnosis. Cryptococci are also sometimes grown from blood culture. *Histoplasma* and *Coccidioides* may also be grown from blood culture in disseminated disease, but are not present in the UK.

3.14   D: Continue all medication and repeat liver function tests in one week

A degree of hepatitis is almost invariable with TB medication but it is rarely a clinical problem. Rifampicin, isoniazid and pyrazinamide are all hepatotoxic. (Ethambutol causes optic neuritis.) The British Thoracic Society recommendations for the treatment of tuberculosis suggest continuing therapy and weekly monitoring of patients if the transaminases are between two and five times the upper limit of normal. TB medication should be discontinued if the transaminases are above five times the upper limit of normal, and gradually re-introduced when the liver function tests have improved. It is important not to undertreat TB or to use a single agent as that increases the likelihood of treatment failure and the development of drug resistance.

3.15   D: Enhanced antimycobacterial immune reaction

This lady has developed an immune reconstitution inflammatory syndrome (IRIS). It is commonly seen and is probably due to recovery of the immune system (due to the antiretrovirals) to a level where the immune system is able to recognise antigens of infectious agents that it had previously failed to recognise. It usually presents with painful enlargement of lymph nodes in the case of TB or *Mycobacterium avium-intracellulare* infection and is associated with fever and an increase in inflammatory markers. (IRIS can occur to antigens of other organisms, eg CMV.) Once the clinician is confident that there is no other infection, it is usually treated with a low dose of steroids.

3.16   A: Request sequencing of his HIV to look for mutations indicating resistance to antiretroviral drugs

It is likely that this man's HIV has developed resistance mutations to his current antiretroviral regime. Detection of resistance mutations by sequencing is now routine practice and is strongly recommended to guide any change of medication in a patient failing therapy, rather than attempting a best guess. Adding a single new agent is bound to fail as restance will develop extremely rapidly. Poor compliance with therapy is more likely to lead to the development of resistant virus. It is always worth rechecking the CD4 count and HIV viral load as the these assays are sometimes subject to laboratory error. His CD4 count is less than $200 \times 10^6/l$. He is therefore at risk of developing *Pneumocystis carinii* pneumonia and should be started on prophylactic co-trimoxazole, but prophylaxis against MAI is not routinely given if the CD4 count is greater than $100 \times 10^6/l$. The measurement of p24 antigen has no place in routine monitoring – it is merely a less sensitive way than RT-PCR of detecting the presence of virus.

3.17   B: bone marrow aspirate

The differential diagnosis is quite wide and includes tuberculosis, lymphoma, HIV and visceral leishmaniasis (kala-azar). (Southern Sudan has been experiencing a continuing epidemic of visceral leishmaniasis for over 15 years.) A bone marrow aspirate will allow culture for TB and leishmaniasis and microscopy for lymphoma, TB and leishmaniasis and will probably give more information than any of the other tests. A liver biopsy (transjugular in view of the thrombocytopenia) would also probably help, but would be less good for the diagnosis of leishmaniasis. Mantoux testing is insensitive in very ill patients (high false-negative rate) and rarely helpful in this situation. Slit skin smears are used for diagnosing cutaneous leishmaniasis and leprosy.

3.18   A: Parvovirus B19

Parvovirus B19 causes a chronic anaemia in immunocompromised patients by causing a persistent infection affecting the erythroblasts. It is spread by the respiratory route and is associated with respiratory symptoms but has only rarely been reported to be associated with any major respiratory problems. It responds to intravenous immunoglobulin, which may have to be given repeatedly in patients who fail to eradicate it due to their immunocompromised state.

3.19   B: Quinine

The patient shoud receive intravenous quinine as soon as possible. Atovaquone/proguanil combination therapy is appropriate for uncomplicated, non-severe *Plasmodium falciparum*. (Artemether and artesunate are at least as effective as quinine in the treatment of falciparum malaria and are in use in areas of quinine resistance in combination with other antimalarial drugs.) Exchange transfusion is suggested for patients with a parasitaemia of more than 30% (or more than 10% with complications) but it has never been subjected to a randomised controlled trial and evidence of efficacy has been obtained from retrospective studies and case reports. Haemofiltration, along with other supportive care is appropriate for established renal failure. *Plasmodium falciparum* malaria resistance to chloroquine is now worldwide and chloroquine should therefore never be used as a treatment option in the UK.

3.20   B: Leptospirosis

The combination of renal failure, jaundice without liver failure and a haemorrhagic conjunctivitis is highly suggestive of leptospirosis (acquired through direct water contact). Deaths tend to occur from myocarditis, overwhelming pulmonary haemorrhage and the complications of renal failure. Scrub typhus causes a debilitating fever and rash, sometimes with CNS involvement. Melioidosis is an extremely common, typical Gram-negative septicaemic illness in the Far East and is acquired through water contact. (It can also cause a more prolonged, less severe illness.) Malaria must always be excluded in any traveller returning from an endemic area, but much of Thailand, including the main tourist areas but excepting the Thai borders, is free of malaria.

3.21   A: Acute HBV infection

Hepatitis B surface antigen (HBsAg) is an early indicator of acute infection. If it persists for more than six months in the presence of IgG antibodies to the core (anti-HBc IgG) it would suggest a chronic carrier state. Antibodies to HbsAg indicate recovery and immunity and are found after successful immunisation.

Anti-HBc IgM appear early in infection and persist during acute infection. The IgG subclass persists for life and indicates previous exposure to the hepatitis B virus.

The 'e' antigen is associated with infectivity and is usually present for three to six weeks, rising and falling within the time span of a raised HbsAg. A persistent 'e' antigen would suggest a chronic carrier status.

3.22   E: Rotavirus

The options are all examples of human RNA viruses. Rotavirus infection occurs mainly in childhood and is associated with respiratory symptoms and diarrhoea. Arboviruses include yellow fever and dengue; arena viruses, Lassa fever and epidemic haemorrhagic fever. Picornavirus is associated with haemorrhagic conjunctivitis. An atypical form of measles, a paramyxovirus, is associated with severe illness and haemorrhage.

3.23   D: Melarsoprol is effective treatment

African trypanosomiasis follows the bite of the tsetse fly and the transfer of *T. brucei*. Humans are an important reservoir for the protozoan. The Rhodesian and Gambian forms of the disease are similar clinically except that Rhodesian sleeping sickness tends to be acute and severe rather than chronic and indolent, and death from Rhodesian disease often occurs within one year. Fever, lymphadenopathy, hepato-splenomegaly, and CNS disease are common features. Suramin and pentamidine are useful therapies but do not cross the blood–brain barrier. CNS disease is best treated with melarsoprol but it is not effective in Rhodesian sleeping sickness.

3.24   B: *Plasmodium falciparum*

In humans, the malaria life cycle starts with the injection of the infective sporozoite through the skin by the *Anopheles* mosquito. During pre-erythrocytic schizogony sporozoites mature to micromerozoites in the liver and are then liberated into the bloodstream and infect red blood cells. It is in the ensuing erythrocytic stage that micromerozoites transform through a trophozoite and shizont phase to become the 'asexual' merozoites that are typically seen on a blood film. Some of these merozoites develop into 'sexual' gametocytes and at this stage the patient becomes infective.

A fourth exoerythrocytic phase exists. This occurs in the liver. A variable number of original sporozoites remain latent in the liver, not transforming to micromerozoites. In this way there appears to be a cycle of continuous re-infection. This phenomenon is definitely seen with *P. vivax*, probably occurs with *P. ovale*, and possibly occurs with *P. malariae*. It is not a feature of the life cycle of *P. falciparum*. It is for this reason that primaquine is required for the eradication of *P. vivax*, *P. ovale*, and *P. malariae*, as it has an effect on the exoerythrocytic cycle.

3.25   A: Cysticercosis

Cysticercosis occurs after ingesting the eggs of *Taenia solium* (pork tapeworm). It is seen in areas of Asia, Africa and South America. Cysterci may develop in any tissue of the body but are most commonly found as space-occupying cerebral lesions and subcutaneous nodules. Retinitis, uveitis, conjunctivitis, choroidal atrophy and blindness may also occur. The treatment of choice is praziquantel.

3.26   D: The Weil–Felix reaction is positive

Q fever is caused by the rickettsia-like organism *Coxiella burnetii*. Although the Weil–Felix agglutination test is being replaced by a complement-fixation test, it is still useful. The test relies on the presence of a common antigen found on some *Rickettsia* and on *Proteus* species. It is positive in the typhus fevers but negative in rickettsial pox, trench fever, and Q fever.

Coxiella burnetii is widespread in domestic and farm animals and is spread by a host tick. Modes of spread to man are thought to include cow's milk, aerosol and dust.

There is usually a fever with a flu-like illness that may resolve or progress to pneumonia or endocarditis. Epididymo-orchitis, uveitis and osteomyelitis have also been documented. Tetracycline is the treatment of choice.

3.27   B: All of the options

Any impairment of host immunity, including chronic alcohol abuse, may add to the risk of an atypical infection. Healthy adults are usually immune, having developed capsular and specific bacterial-related antibodies, either directly related to *Haemophilus* exposure or through cross-reactivity with other common Gram-negative bacteria.

3.28   D: Leptospirosis

Infectious mononucleosis should be considered but the clinical features and risk associated with occupation point towards the spirochaetal infection, leptospirosis (Weil's disease). The early, leptospiraemic phase is characterised by constitutional symptoms of fever, malaise, weight loss, and headache. Infrequently there may be a rash, lymphadenopathy, or hepatosplenomegaly. During the second phase of the infection 50% of patients complain of meningism. Most cases will resolve spontaneously but a small number develop renal impairment, haematuria, haemolytic anaemia, jaundice and cardiac failure.

The organism can be cultured from blood or cerebrospinal fluid in the first week. Serological tests for IgM antibodies are useful. Penicillin or erythromycin are suitable treatments.

3.29   D: None of the options

Epidermolytic toxins of *S. aureus* cause scalded skin syndrome. This is indistinguishable from toxic epidermal necrolysis, which has a number of additional causes. However, given the number of staphylococcal infections, the association is uncommon. Toxic shock syndrome is mediated by toxins TSST1 and enterotoxins B and C; bacteraemia is rare and treatment is mainly supportive, though antibiotics are required to eradicate the focal source. A rapid onset of septicaemia is an infrequent complication of streptococcal cellulitis. Group A β-haemolytic *Streptococcus pyogenes* is associated with erysipelas in the elderly. Impetigo is usually superficial, not affecting the dermis. Ecthyma is an ulcerating form of impetigo, extending into the dermis. Both forms are associated with increased risk of glomerulonephritis.

3.30   A: All of the options

Atypical infections might also include *Nocardia, Candida, Mycoplasma, Mycobacterium,* cytomegalovirus, *Aspergillus,* and *Pneumocystis.*

3.31   D: *Staphylococcus aureus* endocarditis and septicaemia

This is a description of *Staphylococcus aureus* septicaemia, tricuspid endocarditis and septic pulmonary emboli in an intravenous drug user. Confusion is common in severe sepsis and does not always indicate intracranial infection, although this must always be considered. *Streptococcus bovis* endocarditis would typically be less acute, and is associated with underlying gastrointestinal disease (especially bowel cancer) rather than intravenous drug use.

3.32   C: Clarithromycin

Macrolides such as erythromycin and clarithromycin interfere with bacterial ribosomal function. The β-lactam agents, such as amoxicillin, and glycopeptides, such as vancomycin, act by inhibiting cell wall synthesis. The fluoroquinolone ciprofloxacin inhibits bacterial DNA supercoiling by acting on DNA gyrase and topoisomerase enzymes. Trimethoprim is a diaminopyrimidine that acts by inhibiting folic acid synthesis.

3.33   A: *Listeria monocytogenes*

Neonates, the elderly and immunocompromised individuals are at increased risk of *Listeria* meningitis. Pregnant women are prone to listerial bacteraemia, but meningitis is rare; the baby rather than the mother is at risk of central nervous system infection. Amoxicillin or benzylpenicillin are the treatments of choice in listerial meningitis. Cephalosporins are not effective. The CSF findings in listerial meningitis are often only mildly abnormal. The glucose level may be normal, a lymphocytic picture may predominate, and the Gram stain is often negative; a partially treated meningitis of any cause could have similar CSF findings.

3.34   C: Nephritis

CMV infection in HIV-positive individuals (and other immunocompromised patients) is associated with a large variety of presentations. Important manifestations include nervous system infection (retinitis, encephalitis, polyradiculopathy, myelitis), gastrointestinal disease (oesophagitis, colitis, acalculous cholecystitis, hepatitis) and pulmonary involvement (interstitial pneumonitis – much less of a problem in HIV infection than in post-transplant patients). Although urinary shedding of CMV occurs in viraemic patients, CMV nephritis has not been recognised as a significant complication of infection.

3.35   A: CCR5

The gp120, gag and gap-pol gene products, and protease enzyme are all viral products rather than host derived. Gp120 is the viral ligand for the host CD4. CD8 is not involved in HIV attachment. CCR5 is now recognised to be a crucial co-receptor in the HIV replication cycle. Mutations of the gene that codes for this co-receptor have been shown to be protective against HIV infection.

3.36   E: Schistosomiasis

Schistosomiasis usually presents as a chronic disease, typically with liver (principally *Schistosoma mansoni*, *S. japonicum*), bowel (*S. mansoni*, *S. japonicum*) or urinary tract (*S. haematobium*) involvement. However, acute schistosomiasis (Katayama fever) may also occur. The clinical picture in acute schistosomiasis is dominated by allergic phenomena, including fever, urticaria, marked eosinophilia, diarrhoea, hepatosplenomegaly and wheeze.

Amoebiasis and visceral leishmaniasis might explain the diarrhoea and hepatosplenomegaly respectively, but not the wheeze, urticaria and eosinophilia.

3.37   B: JC virus

This is a clinical picture suggestive of the demyelinating disease, progressive multifocal leukoencephalopathy (PML), caused by the JC virus. It typically presents over a period of weeks with focal weakness, slurring of speech, gait disturbance and changes in mental state. Patients are generally afebrile, and CSF analysis is usually normal, though polymerase chain reaction (PCR) assays for JC virus may be positive. Imaging with MRI reveals focal or diffuse white matter lesions that do not enhance with contrast or display mass effect.

The other pathogens listed can cause CNS infection, but none fits the overall clinical scenario as well as JC virus. *Cryptococcus neoformans* and *Mycobacterium tuberculosis* would typically cause a subacute meningitis (with CSF abnormalities), whilst single or multiple ring-enhancing lesions are seen in cerebral toxoplasmosis. *Nocardia asteroides* is a rare cause of brain abscess in the immunocompromised.

3.38   D: Toxic shock syndrome

Not every patient who presents with vomiting and diarrhoea has got gastro-enteritis! The clinical picture here is a classic one for staphylococcal toxic shock syndrome (TSS). The criteria required for a diagnosis of TSS are:

Temperature ≥ 38.5 °C

Hypotension (systolic blood pressure < 90 mmHg)

Rash with subsequent desquamation, particularly on palms and soles

Involvement of at least three of the following organ/systems:

Gastrointestinal (diarrhoea, vomiting)

Musculoskeletal (severe myalgia or raised CPK)

Mucous membranes (hyperaemia of conjunctivae, pharynx or vagina)

Renal (renal impairment)

Hepatic (abnormal liver function tests)

Thrombocytopenia

CNS (disorientation without focal neurology).

Other conditions must also be excluded (eg measles).

3.39   C: Genital herpes

The description is typical of genital herpes, probably HSV-2. His country of origin is irrelevant in this case. If he entered the UK recently, then 'exotic' STDs such as chancroid and LGV would need to be considered, but the clinical presentation is not suggestive of either of these. Syphilis (painless, smooth ulcers) must always be considered in genital ulcer disease, but again the clinical picture does not fit with this or with Behçet's disease.

3.40   E: Toxic side-effects of isoniazid are best reduced by the concomitant use of rifabutin

Rifampicin, isoniazid, ethambutol, rifabutin, and pyrazinamide are commonly used antituberculous drugs. Rifampicin and isoniazid may cause hepatitis. The toxic effects of isoniazid also include peripheral neuritis and lupus-like symptoms, and can be reduced by the concomitant use of pyrazinamide. Rifabutin causes uveitis and the risk of this is raised by the concomitant use of macrolide antibiotics or triazole antifungals. The dose of rifabutin should be reduced in this situation. Capreomycin is reserved for drug-resistant cases and is associated with nephrotoxicity, ototoxicity, hepatitis and eosinophilia.

4.1 E: Persistence of rheumatoid factor at high titre is a risk factor for the development of rheumatoid arthritis

Around 70% of all patients with established rheumatoid arthritis and up to 100% of patients with nodules are seropositive for IgM rheumatoid factor. However, the prevalence is much lower at disease onset and it is found in other connective tissue diseases, in response to infection (particularly chronic infection), and the prevalence is increased in the elderly (up to 30% in some series). Presence of rheumatoid factor is the best predictor of erosive outcome, identified to date, in rheumatoid arthritis. A persistently raised titre has been shown to increase the probability of developing rheumatoid arthritis in the future.

4.2 E: Hyperviscocity syndrome is a recognised complication of therapy with gold salts

Sulfasalazine requires regular blood monitoring, particularly frequently when treatment is initiated because of the risk of agranulocytosis. Methotrexate may cause worsening of rheumatoid nodules. Side-effects of antimalarials include reversible corneal deposits and, very rarely, irreversible bulls-eye maculopathy. D-Penicillamine is associated with a number of drug-induced autoimmune syndromes, including drug-induced lupus. Hypogammaglobulinaemia rather than hyperviscocity is associated with treatment with gold.

4.3 A: If he is found to carry the HLA-B27 antigen the course is more likely to be chronic

The history is suggestive of reactive arthritis secondary to a dysenteric infection. The joint swelling is characteristically sterile and treatment with antibiotics will have no effect on the course of the arthritis. The classic triad is of arthritis, non-gonococcal urethritis and conjunctivitis, but conjunctivitis only occurs in approximately 30% of cases. The sacro-iliac joints may be involved and this can be unilateral or bilateral. HLA-B27 has prognostic implications because, if present, the arthritis is more likely to become chronic or recurrent.

4.4 C: Dermatomyositis

The history is typical of dermatomyositis with skin involvement manifesting as the shawl sign, with a characteristic distribution involving the face, upper arms and neck. Although photosensitivity is characteristic of SLE, it also occurs in dermatomyositis. ANA is likely to be positive in many connective tissue diseases and therefore will not help in diagnosis. The absence of antibodies to RNP makes a diagnosis of mixed connective tissue disease unlikely, whilst the absence of sclerodactyly or thickened skin makes systemic sclerosis unlikely.

4.5   B: Amyloidosis associated with nephrotic syndrome

Behçet's disease is twice as common in males, with a mean age at onset of 30 years and has its highest prevalence in Turkey, Iran and Japan. The hallmark of disease is aphthous orogenital ulcerations. Erythema nodosum occurs in 50% of cases. Arthritis also affects around 50% of cases and is usually a self-limiting non-deforming, non-erosive, peripheral oligoarthritis. There is no association with B27 carriage or sacro-iliac joint involvement. Neurological complications present with pyramidal, cerebellar or sensory signs. A vasculitis affecting both arteries and veins can occur. Venous thrombosis occurs in about 25% of cases, and arterial occlusion or aneurysms can result in cerebrovascular accidents, hypertension or limb ischaemia. A chronic relapsing bilateral anterior +/– posterior uveitis can cause blindness. The deposition of AA amyloid is a complication of chronic inflammation and usually occurs in the context of nephritic syndrome.

4.6   B: Recurrent episodes of ear swelling that spare the pinna

Relapsing polychondritis is a rare condition characterised by recurrent episodes of cartilage swelling. It typically presents with nasal or ear involvement but the lobule is spared (unlike infection, which involves the lobule). Recurrent inflammation of the cartilage results in weakness and can cause a saddle-nose deformity, floppy ears and respiratory symptoms due to laryngotracheal strictures. A seronegative, asymmetrical, non-erosive arthritis develops in around 75% of cases. Scleritis, iritis, and cardiac complications may also occur. Treatment options include non-steroidal anti-inflammatory drugs (NSAIDs), colchicine or steroids.

4.7   D: Polyarteritis nodosa (PAN)

Wegener's can affect the eyes, ENT and upper respiratory tract, lower respiratory tract and kidneys, and involve the peripheral or central nervous systems. However, vasculitis involving the gastrointestinal tract is uncommon. Microscopic polyangiitis primarily affects the kidneys, and Churg–Strauss syndrome is associated with atopy, peripheral neuropathy, eosinophilia and fleeting pulmonary granuloma. Both Henoch–Schönlein vasculitis and PAN can involve the gastrointestinal tract, kidneys and skin but PAN is more commonly associated with a peripheral neuropathy. Henoch–Schönlein vasculitis can occur in adults but is much commoner in children.

4.8   C: Osteoarthritis (OA) is the most likely diagnosis

Hyperuricaemia is ten times more common than gout and uric acid levels can be normal during a flare-up of gout. Hence, uric acid can neither confirm nor exclude a diagnosis of gout in this case where joint pain is current. Similarly, chondrocalcinosis (presence of calcium in the joint) is much more common than pseudogout and the commonest joints involved are the knees, wrists and index metacarpal joints (haemochromatosis). OA commonly affects the first MTP joint and, until the diagnosis is confirmed, treatment with allopurinol should not be commenced. In the absence of a positive family history, a history of alcohol excess or other medication, OA is more likely than gout.

4.9   B: ESR

In this age group, polymyalgia rheumatica (PMR) is much more likely than myositis as a cause of difficulty lifting the arms above the head. Movement is restricted due to stiffness in PMR as opposed to weakness in myositis. Muscle biopsies and creatinine kinase can be normal in myositis, particularly dermatomyositis. While the ESR will be high in myositis, it will be very high in PMR and, therefore, this is the best test.

4.10   E: Osteoporosis is diagnosed when the T score is ≤ –2.5

Not all treatments are effective in all patients, so it is wise to obtain baseline bone density readings to enable you to monitor the effectiveness of the osteoprotection. Etidronate is used as prophylaxis for steroid-induced osteoporosis but is complicated to take and may not be the best choice for an elderly lady. All trials of bisphosphonates have used calcium supplementation and, especially as this lady is immobile and elderly, there may be some co-existing osteomalacia. Results of bone density scanning should be compared to the peak bone mass (T score) rather than to an age-matched control (Z score).

4.11   C: ACE inhibitors should be introduced as soon as any rise in blood pressure is noted

The fact that this lady has tight skin which includes her upper arms indicates that she has diffuse systemic sclerosis (dSSc) rather than limited cutaneous (lcSSc), where skin involvement is limited to the hands and forearms, the head and neck and the legs and feet. Trials of penicillamine in treating the skin changes of systemic sclerosis have been disappointing. The commonest cause of death in dSSc is pulmonary fibrosis. Pulmonary hypertension does occur in around 5% of cases but is more common as a late complication of lcSSc (CREST) (~ 25% cases). ANA may be positive in many connective tissue diseases. A serious complication of dSSc is scleroderma renal crisis, which is associated with renal failure and death. The introduction of ACE inhibitors at an early stage can preserve renal function and avert this complication.

4.12 C: Oligoarthritis affecting the lower limbs, associated with bilateral hilar lymphadenopathy and erythema nodosum

The most common form of joint involvement in sarcoidosis is an arthropathy affecting particularly the large joints of the lower limb, often associated with bilateral hilar lymphadenopathy, erythema nodosum, uveitis or lupus pernio. The joints are affected in a symmetrical manner and the arthropathy can last for weeks to months. Erythema chronicum migrans is characteristic of Lyme disease.

4.13 B: Arthritis of the distal interphalangeal (DIP) joints is usually associated with nail involvement

Psoriatic arthritis (PsA) is an inflammatory arthritis associated with psoriasis and usually negative for rheumatoid factor. However, the presence of RF does not exclude the diagnosis. The commonest presentation is with an oligoarthritis affecting the large joints of the lower limbs but DIP joint involvement is the classic presentation and is almost always associated with nail involvement. The prevalence of HLA-B27 is higher in PsA, particularly in those with sacro-iliac joint involvement. However, B27 is also found in the normal population and cannot, therefore, be used to confirm the diagnosis. There is a risk of antimalarials exacerbating skin psoriasis but they can be used to treat the arthritis. Acute anterior uveitis is the characteristic ocular manifestation.

4.14 B: *Staphylococcus aureus*

Staphylococcus aureus accounts for over 50% of infection and β-haemolytic *Streptococcus* around 10%. In children under two years of age *Haemophilus* is common. Lower limbs tend to be affected more than upper limbs. In children the commonest site is the hips while the knee is involved more often in adults. *Neisseria gonorrhoeae* is a cause of septic arthritis in young adults and is often associated with painless skin lesions. Lyme disease is caused by the spirochaete *Borrelia burgdorferi*. It presents with erythema marginatum at the site of the tick bite, arthritis (recurrent brief attacks), neurological (lymphocytic meningitis, encephalomyelitis) and cardiac (second/third-degree AV conduction defects) complications.

4.15   C: Chronic anterior iridocyclitis

The iris and ciliary body both form the anterior uveal tract. Therefore, iridocyclitis is anterior uveitis. Chronic asymptomatic anterior uveitis is a well-recognised complication of juvenile idiopathic arthritis, particular the pauciarticular forms. It is bilateral in two-thirds of cases and therefore regular slit lamp screening examinations are required as it may lead to blindness. Acute anterior uveitis is characteristic of the seronegative spondyloarthropathies, while conjunctivitis occurs in Reiter's/reactive arthritis. Scleritis occurs in rheumatoid arthritis, SLE, Wegener's granulomatosis and other forms of vasculitis. Posterior uveitis occurs in Behçet's disease, Wegener's granulomatosis and sarcoidosis.

4.16   B: Any of these items

Non-steroidal anti-inflammatory drugs (NSAIDs) may interact with a number of different medications. Methotrexate and lithium levels may rise. Although a recognised interaction, it is very common to find patients on both methotrexate and an NSAID. Monitoring of the full blood count and liver function every four to six weeks is essential with methotrexate treatment, whether taking NSAIDs or not.

The effectiveness of thiazides, loop diuretics, β-blockers, ACE inhibitors, and oral hypoglycaemic agents may fall. There is also an increased risk of hyperkaleamia with potassium-sparing diuretics.

The patient is also taking corticosteroids. This may increase the risk of gastro-intestinal bleeding and exacerbate fluid retention.

4.17   C: Use of a β-blocker

Men over the age of 60 years may lose bone density, but the risk of osteoporotic fracture does not appear to increase in men until after the age of 70. Other risk factors include hypogonadism (low testosterone levels), smoking, chronic alcohol abuse, lack of exercise, poor nutrition, drugs (such as corticosteroids, heparin, thyroxine, and phenytoin), and disorders such as rheumatoid arthritis, diabetes mellitus, chronic liver or renal disease, malabsorption syndromes, and endocrinopathies (Cushing's syndrome, hyperthyroidism, hyperparathyroidism). Low-trauma fractures should be investigated with dual energy X-ray absorptiometry (DEXA) at all ages, though there is an argument for commencing the elderly patient (> 80 years) on calcium and vitamin D without scanning, and/or newer bisphosphonates in the presence of new spinal fractures.

4.18   C: Drugs implicated in the aetiology of DIL should not be used in idiopathic systemic lupus erythematosus

Many drugs have been implicated in causing drug-induced lupus (DIL). Those definitely and most commonly associated with DIL are hydralazine, procainamide, isoniazid, quinidine, methyldopa, chlorpromazine, and salazopyrin. Hydralazine-associated DIL is considered to be dose-dependent, and procainamide time-dependent. Up to 90% of patients taking procainamide develop a positive antinuclear antibody (ANA) and 30% of these develop DIL.

Renal, central nervous system and skin features of systemic lupus erythematosus (SLE) are rare in DIL. Other features of SLE, such as articular, pulmonary and serosal disease are common.

In the majority of cases the condition subsides on withdrawing the drug. There is no contraindication to using these drugs in idiopathic SLE.

4.19   A: All of the options

The granular, diffuse and cytoplasm-distributed cANCA affects the target antigen proteinase 3 and is associated with Wegener's granulomatosis. The perinuclear-distributed pANCA binds to several enzymes, including myeloperoxidase, and is associated with microscopic polyangiitis, polyarteritis nodosa, Churg–Strauss syndrome, Felty's syndrome and inflammatory bowel disease. An atypical perinuclear aANCA is found in inflammatory bowel diseases, endocarditis, and HIV.

4.20   A: A skin biopsy often demonstrates evidence of vasculitis

These features are consistent with familial Mediterranean fever (FMF), though the differential diagnosis might include polyarteritis nodosa, porphyria, hereditary angio-oedema, rheumatic fever, or septic arthritis.

FMF is an autosomal recessive disorder. The genetic defect is on chromosome 16. Most cases (80%) present before the age of 20 years and most frequently in people of eastern Mediterranean descent (Armenians, Arabs and Sephardic and Ashkenazi Jews).

Serositis is common: 95% of cases have abdominal attacks and 50% pleural attacks. Arthritis occurs in 75% of cases and an erysipelas-like rash in up to 50% of cases. There may be erosive joint disease and the most common picture is a monoarthritis. This tends to resolve spontaneously over weeks to months. The skin lesions show a dermal infiltration of neutrophils rather than a vasculitis.

Amyloidosis can occur in up to 40% of cases, leading to renal failure, proteinuria, or malabsorption. An elevated ESR, leucocytosis, normochromic normocytic anaemia, and inflammatory synovial fluid are all non-specific features. Colchicine may help. Corticosteroids are unhelpful.

4.21 D: Joint pains in more than one joint for one week

Hypermobility is considered present if a person satisfies four or more manoeuvres in the nine-point Beighton hypermobility score:

The ability to:	R	L
1. Passively dorsiflex the 5th metacarpophalangeal joint to $\geq 90°$	1	1
2. Oppose the thumb to the volar aspect of the ipsilateral forearm	1	1
3. Hyperextend the elbow $\geq 10°$	1	1
4. Hyperextend the knee $\geq 10°$	1	1
5. Place hands flat on the floor without bending the knees		1
Total score		9

Other joints, not included in this scoring system, may also be hypermobile and specialists in this area will take them into account when considering a diagnosis of hypermobility. Likewise, a history of being able to do these manoeuvres in the past is important when examining older patients whose levels of flexibility may now be reduced. Benign joint hypermobility syndrome (BJHS) is excluded in the presence of Marfan's or Ehlers–Danlos syndrome. The revised (Beighton 1988) criteria for BJHS are shown below. BJHS is diagnosed in the presence of two major, one major and two minor, or four minor criteria. Two minor criteria will suffice where there is an unequivocally affected first-degree relative.

Major criteria:

1. A Beighton score of 4/9 or greater (either current or historical)
2. Arthralgia for longer than three months in four or more joints.

Minor criteria:

1. A Beighton score of 1, 2 or 3/9
2. Arthralgia in one to three joints or back pain, either for longer than three months, spondylosis/spondylolisthesis
3. Dislocation/subluxation in more than one joint, or one joint on more than one occasion
4. Soft tissue rheumatism in three or more sites
5. Marfanoid habitus
6. Abnormal skin: striae, hyperextensibility, papyraceous scars
7. Eye signs: drooping eyelids, myopia, antimongoloid slant
8. Varicose veins, herniae, uterine/rectal prolapse.

4.22   B: Serum uric acid levels are increased in Fanconi's syndrome

Increased levels of serum uric acid are seen in states of high purine turnover or reduced renal excretion. High purine turnover states include lympho- and myeloproliferative disorders, chemotherapy, psoriasis, haemolytic anaemia, and pregnancy. Reduced renal clearance may occur in renal failure, with the use of diuretics (except spironolactone), low-dose salicylates, ciclosporin, ethambutol, pyrazinamide, alcohol, metabolic acidosis, hypothyroidism, hypo- and hyper-parathyroidism, and lead poisoning.

Uricosuric drugs reduce serum levels of uric acid. These include probenecid and high-dose salicylates. Fanconi's syndrome and Wilson's disease are both associated with decreased levels of serum uric acid.

Inherited metabolic syndromes of hyperuricaemia include Lesch–Nyhan syndrome (X-linked hypoxanthine guanine phosphoribosyl transferase deficiency) and von Gierke's disease (autosomal recessive glucose-6-phosphatase deficiency).

4.23   D: Systemic lupus erythematosus

Autoantibodies to dsDNA are found in up to 60% of cases of systemic lupus erythematosus (SLE). The antibody is associated with nephritis and severe disease. The Sm autoantibody is found in up to 40% of cases and associated with interstitial lung disease. It is very uncommon to find these autoantibodies in association with other autoimmune rheumatic diseases.

Autoantibodies to snRNP are also common in SLE, but are less specific and may be found in overlap syndromes with features of polymyositis and systemic sclerosis. Anti-Ro and anti-La antibodies may be found in 10–30% of SLE patients. They are, however, more commonly associated with Sjögren's syndrome.

Less than 5% of patients with SLE will have Scl-70 autoantibodies (indicative of diffuse systemic sclerosis), centromere autoantibodies (indicative of limited scleroderma), or Jo-1 autoantibodies (suggestive of poly/dermatomyositis).

4.24   A: All of the options

All of the options are associated with aggressive disease in rheumatoid arthritis. Other features include an elevated ESR, bony erosions on plain X-rays, and multiple joint involvement.

4.25   E: Start the patient on 60 mg/day oral prednisolone

Temporal arteritis, often associated with polymyalgia rheumatica, tends to occur abruptly and is commonly associated with either a temporal or occipital headache, scalp tenderness, constitutional symptoms, jaw claudication, and visual disturbance. In the presence of the latter, high-dose oral prednisolone should be commenced immediately to try and prevent visual loss from ischaemic optic neuropathy. A high ESR and histological evidence of arteritis are useful diagnostic tests. Although a biopsy is best performed as early as possible, the introduction of prednisolone should never be delayed.

The dose of steroid can be tapered downwards slowly in steps of 5–10 mg every two to four weeks according to symptom control and a falling ESR. When the daily dose has reached 10 mg/day it is advised that a slower tapering regime be employed at 1-mg reductions every two weeks. Most patients will require daily maintenance doses of approximately 5 mg for 12 to 24 months. Some cases require longer-term and higher-dose maintenance therapy. In cases where this seems likely (prednisolone dose ≥ 7.5 mg/day for three months) prophylaxis against corticosteroid-induced osteoporosis should be started.

4.26   D: Measure spirochaete antibodies

Lyme disease (LD) is a spirochaete (*Borrelia burgdorferi*) tick-borne infection common throughout the world and in particular northern USA. The hallmark of LD is an annular erythematous and often large (> 20 cm) rash (erythema chronicum migrans (ECM)) at the site of the tick bite. However, many people do not recall the bite or the rash. Constitutional symptoms of fever and fatigue may precede headaches, myalgia, arthralgia, tendonopathy, conjunctivitis, uveitis, pharyngitis, lymphadenopathy and testicular swelling.

Weeks later there may be cardiac or neurological symptoms and months later there may be a persistent inflammatory arthropathy and an atrophic rash of acrodermatitis chronica atrophicans.

Raised IgG or specific IgM antibodies to the spirochaete can be found two to four weeks after infection. The diagnosis is clinical, supported by this serological test.

Early disease is best treated with amoxicillin, doxycycline, or clarithromycin. Later cardiac, neurological, or persistent arthritic symptoms may also require a cephalosporin.

4.27   E: Warfarin should be dosed to maintain the INR at 2.0

Antiphospholipid syndrome is associated with recurrent venous and arterial thrombosis, spontaneous abortion, vasculitis, CNS disorders, and a 'catastrophic' widespread organ failure. Thrombocytopenia is seen in up to 25% of cases.

Antibodies are found in 5% of the general population and in association with several autoimmune rheumatic diseases (especially SLE), vasculitides, infection, and malignancy. Both the lupus anticoagulant and anticardiolipin antibodies should be measured though one and not the other may be present in up to 40% of cases. The lupus anticoagulant cannot be measured if the patient is already on heparin or warfarin.

Recurrent thrombosis should be treated with high-dose warfarin at an INR of 3–4.

4.28   C: Hypothyroidism

The following are recognised causes of ectopic calcification: hyperparathyroidism, hyperphosphataemia, sarcoidosis, hypervitaminosis D, tumour lysis, dermato-myositis, scleroderma.

Ossification of soft tissues occurs most often following traumatic myositis.

4.29   A: Churg–Strauss syndrome

Other rheumatic diseases associated with pyoderma gangrenosum include systemic lupus erythematosus, Wegener's granulomatosis and sarcoidosis. Diabetes, haematological diseases such as leukaemia and myelofibrosis, and gastrointestinal disorders, including inflammatory bowel disease, chronic active hepatitis and primary biliary cirrhosis are also associated with the condition.

4.30   E: Raised parathyroid hormone

Pseudohypoparathyroidism (PHP) occurs as a result of target tissue resistance to parathyroid hormone (PTH). The biochemical consequences are hypocalcaemia, hyperphosphataemia and a raised PTH.

Pseudohypoparathyroidism may be tested for by measuring urine excretion of cyclic AMP (cAMP) in response to PTH. Administration of PTH to normal individuals leads to increased urinary excretion of cAMP. An abnormal response to this test in individuals with PHP classifies them as either type I (no increase in urine cAMP) or type II (normal increase in urine cAMP but abnormal renal phosphate handling).

The clinical features of PHT include short stature, round facies, obesity, and brachydactyly. Pseudopseudohypoparathyroidism describes the clinical features in the presence of a normal serum calcium and PTH/cAMP test.

REVISION CHECKLISTS

CLINICAL PHARMACOLOGY: REVISION CHECKLIST

Interactions/dose adjustment

- [ ] Drug interactions
- [ ] Pregnancy/breastfeeding
- [ ] Adverse effects – general
- [ ] Dose adjustment in renal failure
- [ ] Drugs in porphyria
- [ ] Polymorphism of drug metabolism
- [ ] Overdose/poisoning

Specific side-effects of drugs

- [ ] Asthma exacerbation
- [ ] Drugs causing hypothyroidism
- [ ] Gynaecomastia/hyperprolactinaemia
- [ ] Hepatic enzyme inducers
- [ ] Hypokalaemia
- [ ] Aggravation of skin disorders
- [ ] Convulsions
- [ ] Haemolytic anaemia

Fundamental pharmacology

- [ ] Mechanisms of drug/antibiotic action

Most frequently considered individual agents

- [ ] Antipsychotics/depressants
- [ ] ACE inhibitors
- [ ] Amiodarone
- [ ] Thiazides
- [ ] Anticonvulsants
- [ ] Digoxin
- [ ] Lithium
- [ ] Sulfasalazine

- [ ] Metronidazole
- [ ] Radio-iodine

Other 'topical' agents

- [ ] Azidothymidine (AZT)
- [ ] Antihypertensives
- [ ] Cimetidine
- [ ] Gentamicin
- [ ] Griseofulvin
- [ ] HMG Co-A reductase inhibitor
- [ ] Immunosuppressants
- [ ] L-dopa
- [ ] Metronidazole
- [ ] Nitrates
- [ ] NSAIDs
- [ ] Penicillamine
- [ ] Retinoic acid
- [ ] Warfarin

IMMUNOLOGY: REVISION CHECKLIST

Cytokines

- ☐ Tumour necrosis factor
- ☐ Interferon
- ☐ Inflammatory mediators (general)
- ☐ Leukotrienes

Cellular immunity

- ☐ T lymphocytes/deficiency
- ☐ Cell-mediated immunity

Immunoglobulins/autoimmunity

- ☐ IgA/IgE/IgG
- ☐ Autoimmune disease/ANCA
- ☐ Hypogammaglobulinaemia
- ☐ Monoclonal gammopathy
- ☐ Tissue receptor antibodies
- ☐ Circulating immune complexes
- ☐ Precipitating antibodies in diagnosis

Miscellaneous

- ☐ Complement/CH_{50}
- ☐ Angioneurotic oedema
- ☐ Hypersensitivity reactions
- ☐ Mast cells
- ☐ Polymerase chain reaction
- ☐ Post-splenectomy
- ☐ Transplant rejection
- ☐ Acute phase reactants

INFECTIOUS DISEASES: REVISION CHECKLIST

Viral infections

- ☐ Hepatitis
- ☐ Infectious mononucleosis
- ☐ Chickenpox/measles/mumps
- ☐ AIDS/HIV
- ☐ Adenovirus
- ☐ Genital herpes
- ☐ Parvovirus

Bacterial infections

- ☐ Venereal disease
- ☐ Brucellosis
- ☐ TB/BCG
- ☐ Tetanus
- ☐ Toxoplasmosis
- ☐ Typhoid/cholera
- ☐ *Bacteroides*
- ☐ *Haemophilus influenzae*
- ☐ *Helicobacter pylori*
- ☐ Lyme disease
- ☐ Meningitis
- ☐ Pneumonia
- ☐ *Staphylococcus*
- ☐ Diphtheria

Routes of infection

- ☐ Transmission by insect bite
- ☐ Faecal–oral transmission

Tropical and protozoal infections

- ☐ Malaria
- ☐ Tropical fever/splenomegaly
- ☐ Giardiasis
- ☐ *Pneumocystis carinii*
- ☐ Schistosomiasis

Miscellaneous

- ☐ *Chlamydia trachomatis*
- ☐ Other infections/diarrhoea
- ☐ Chronic infection and anaemia
- ☐ Infections and eosinophilia
- ☐ Prion disease

RHEUMATOLOGY: REVISION CHECKLIST

Autoimmune disease

☐ Rheumatoid arthritis
☐ SLE
☐ Wegener's granulomatosis

Other vasculitides

☐ Polymyalgia rheumatica
☐ Cranial arteritis
☐ Vasculitic disease

Other arthritides

☐ Reiter's syndrome
☐ Ankylosing spondylitis/HLA-B27
☐ Arthralgia
☐ Behçet's disease
☐ Arthropathy (general)
☐ Hypertrophic osteoarthropathy
☐ Osteoarthritis
☐ Pseudogout

Miscellaneous

☐ Antiphospholipid syndrome
☐ Digital gangrene
☐ Peri-articular calcification
☐ Systemic sclerosis

INDEX

Locators refer to question number.

Clinical Pharmacology

Immunology

Infectious Diseases

Rheumatology

PASTEST

PasTest has been established since 1972 and is the leading provider of exam-related medical revision course sand books in the UK. The company has a dedicated customer services team to ensure that doctors can easily get up to date information about our products and to ensure that their orders are dealt with efficiently. Our extensive experience means that we are always one step ahead when it comes to knowledge of the current trends and contents of the Royal College exams.

In the last 12 months we have sold over 67,000 books to medical students and qualified doctors. These may be purchased through bookshops, over the telephone or online at our website. All books are reviewed prior to publication to ensure that they mirror the needs of candidates and therefore act as an invaluable aid to exam preparation.

Test yourself online

PasTest Online is a new database that will be launched this year. With more than 1500 Best of Five questions prepared by experts, PasTest Online:

- enables you to test yourself whenever you want

- is accessible whatever time of day

- is reasonably priced and has excellent exam revision tips

- has a choice of mock exam, random questions and specialist questions. This means that you can test yourself in certain weak areas or take a mock exam.

Interested? Try a free demo at www.pastestonline.co.uk

100% Money Back Guarantee

We're sure you will find our study books invaluable, but in the unlikely event that you are not entirely happy, we will give you your money back – guaranteed.

Delivery to your Door

With a busy lifestyle, nobody enjoys walking to the shops for something that may or may not be in stock. Let us take the hassle and deliver direct to your door. We will despatch your book within 24 hours of receiving your order. We also offer free delivery on books for medical students to UK addresses.

How to Order:

🖥 www.pastest.co.uk

To order books safely and securely online, shop at our website.

☎ Telephone: +44 (0)1565 752000

📠 Fax: +44 (0)1565 650264

✉ PasTest Ltd, FREEPOST, Knutsford, WA16 7BR.